T0251226

THE CRISIS OF COMPETENCE

Transitional Stress and the Displaced Worker

Brunner/Mazel Psychosocial Stress Series
Charles R. Figley, Ph.D., Series Editor

BRUNNER/MAZEL PSYCHOSOCIAL STRESS SERIES No. 16

THE CRISIS OF COMPETENCE

Transitional Stress and the Displaced Worker

Carl A. Maida, PH.D.
Norma S. Gordon, M.A.
Norman L. Farberow, PH.D.

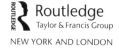 Routledge
Taylor & Francis Group

NEW YORK AND LONDON

To the many individuals whose lives have been changed
by the trauma of job loss

Library of Congress Cataloging-in-Publication Data

Maida, Carl A.
    The crisis of competence: transitional stress and the displaced worker /
Carl A. Maida, Norma S. Gordon, Norman L. Farberow.
        p. cm. — (Brunner/Mazel psychosocial stress series; no. 16)
    Bibliography: p.
    Includes index.
    ISBN 0-87630-559-1
    1. Unemployment—Psychological aspects. 2. Unemployed—Counseling of.
3. Plant shutdowns. I. Gordon, Norma S. II. Farberow, Norman L.
III. Title. IV. Series.
    [DNLM: 1. Community Mental Health Services. 2. Life Change Events.
3. Stress, Psychological—therapy. 4. Unemployment. W1 BR917TB no. 16 /
WM 172 M217c]
    HD5708.M34 1989
331.13'7—dc20
DNLM/DLC
for Library of Congress   89-15825
                                                                     CIP

First published 1989 by BRUNNER\MAZEL, INC.
Philadelphia and London

This edition published 2015 by Routledge
711 Third Avenue, New York, NY 10017, USA
27 Church Road, Hove, East Sussex BN3 2FA

Routledge is an imprint of the Taylor & Francis Group, an informa business

ISBN 13: 978-0-87630-559-1 (hbk)
ISBN 13: 978-1-138-86910-3 (pbk)

Editorial Note

The Editorial Board of the Psychosocial Stress Book Series is proud and delighted to add this fifteenth volume to the Series. This book focuses on a psychosocial stressor that affects thousands and thousands of people every year. The displaced worker is denied the dignity bestowed by employment, in addition to a source of income, security, and insurance benefits. This topic has attracted considerable speculation, but little research and careful analysis. This important volume contains both thorough research and thoughtful interpretations.

As the subscriber to this Series is aware, the Series strives to develop and publish books that in some way make a significant contribution to the understanding and management of the psychosocial stress-reaction paradigm. In particular, Series books are designed to advance the work of clinicians, researchers, and other professionals involved in the varied aspects of human services. These professionals must help clients confront and find solutions to the challenges associated with psychosocial stress.

This book and every book proposed for the Series is subjected to an intensive review by the Editorial Board. This "refereed" book series insures that only the most important contributions are published. Indeed, the quality and significance of the Series are a product of this nationally and internationally respected group of scholars who compose the Editorial Board. Like the readership, the Board represents the fields of general medicine, pediatrics, psychiatry, nursing, psychology, sociology, social work, family therapy, political science, and anthropology.

Books in the Series, such as this one, focus on the stress associated with a wide variety of psychosocial stressors. Collectively, the books and chapters in the series have focused on the immediate and long-term psychosocial consequences of extraordinary stressors such as divorce, parenting, separation, rape, incest, and other crime victimization, racism, social isolation, acute illness, drug addiction, death, sudden unemployment, war, natural disasters, and many others.

We are especially pleased to welcome this book into the Psychosocial Stress Book Series. It provides not only a solid, scientific contribution to the field, but also needed direction for clinical work with displaced workers. Together with this most recent volume, these Series books form a new orientation for thinking about human behavior under extraordinary conditions. They provide an integrated set of source books for scholars and practitioners interested in how and why some individuals and social systems thrive under stressful situations such as job loss and occupational displacement, while others do not.

CHARLES R. FIGLEY, PH.D.
Series Editor
Florida State University
Tallahassee, Florida

Contents

Acknowledgments

We would like to thank Ray Gibson, former President of UAW Local 216, the members of his Executive Committee, other representatives of the United Auto Workers, and Donald Stockman of the State of California Department of Mental Health, for acknowledging the need and supporting the development and funding of a stress counseling program for workers laid off by the closure of the General Motors Assembly Division plant in Southgate, California. In addition, we want to recognize the efforts of the local and state elected officials, the General Motors Corporation executives, and the United Auto Workers that made possible the development of a retraining program that included stress counseling services as a component in this and later federal Job Training Partnership Act Title III programs. We want to thank specifically the City of Los Angeles Community Development Department, the City of Los Angeles Private Industry Council, and the Los Angeles Business Labor Council for their consistent advocacy.

We would like to thank Nanette Levine for bringing her experience in working with labor unions and their members to the development of these innovative counseling programs for displaced workers. We are grateful to Ruth Shelkun of the Washtenaw Community Mental Health Center in Ann Arbor, Michigan, and to Betty Tableman, of the State of Michigan Department of Mental Health, who generously shared materials on the programs developed in that state for displaced workers. Lee Schore and Michael Lerner, of the Institute for Labor and Mental Health, in Oakland, California, shared their research and clinical insights on stress and the workplace. David Dooley, of the University of California, Irvine, encouraged us to document our experiences and generously shared his own research on unemployment and mental health. Charles Roppel, of the State of California Department of Mental Health, shared the innovative health promotion materials developed by his program. Alfred Katz, of the University of California, Los Angeles, was supportive throughout the project and helped provide a historical frame of reference on workplace mental health efforts in this country.

Norman Farberow would like to thank Pearl for her constant encouragement and support, and Nancy Taylor, who typed portions of the manuscript with loyalty and diligence. Norma Gordon expresses her appreciation to her husband, Edwin, for his caring and patience, and to her sons, Peter, Joshua and Alexander for their consistent encouragement, Carl Maida would like to thank his children, Vanessa and Alexandra, for their love and support during the writing of this book.

Foreword

Despite the existence of ameliorative resources such as unemployment insurance and special provisions in collective bargaining contracts, unemployment remains a major source of economic hardship, deprivation, stress, and ill health among working people in many countries.

Unemployment is particularly class-oriented, since blue-collar workers are most massively and seriously affected by it. Thus, in the United States the 1985 unemployment rate for "operators, fabricators, and laborers" was 11.3%, while that for "managers and professionals" was 2.6%.

While the effects of unemployment on individuals and society have been studied especially since the Great Depression of the 1930s (e.g., in the outstanding works of Bakke and Jahoda), some newer phenomena are now associated with it. So-called "structural unemployment" has resulted from the decline of the older "smokestack" industries in the United States—steel, automobile, rubber, and machine tool production. Layoffs as a result of such structural causes and of periodic *under*employment put new strains primarily on the blue-collar, industrial work force, but on white-collar employees as well.

The more recent experience of unemployment in the United States also has produced some stresses for workers and their families to which they were not previously subjected: unpleasant, anxiety-ridden encounters with the government insurance bureaucracy; fears of losing job-related health insurance coverage; and the entry of wives into the labor force in order to keep the household going.

Despite these new elements, however, the impact of unemployment currently is similar to what it has been historically.

Incomes are sharply reduced, since unemployment benefits are well below prevailing wage levels and usually expire after 26 weeks. Families draw on their savings, drastically curtail their levels of expenditure, often cannot meet mortgage or rent payments, and face eviction or foreclosures.

All these stressful economic problems affect the mental and physical health of the unemployed worker and family members to a degree perhaps not experienced in any other common situation, and place them in a vulnerable, high-risk group.

To combat these threats to mental and physical health, some comprehensive and creative projects have been organized. This book gives a remarkably clear and analytical account of some of the most important and successful of these, conducted in Southern California with multiple populations of displaced workers.

The demonstration programs described in this volume involved the close working collaboration of several interests: the trade unions that represented the workers; the corporations that had employed them and were now seeking to lay off, retire, relocate, or dismiss them; and Federal and State agencies concerned with employment and vocational retraining.

To realize their objectives, these projects clearly had to involve the intersectoral cooperation of many public and private agencies, and to include, at a specific local level, the Los Angeles City and County Departments of Health, Housing, Mental Health, Education, and Community Development, as well as local community institutions, churches, schools, hospitals, voluntary health agencies, and their professionals.

The main purpose of the various projects was to meet the post-layoff problems of groups of displaced workers, who participated in jointly sponsored programs of counseling, industrial retraining, and job placement.

The presentation depicts in fascinating detail the obstacles—political, organizational and attitudinal—that made it difficult to achieve cooperation and consensus among the varying interest groups involved. The successful resolution of these differences, as well as the achievement of such broadly conceived, novel programs required community organization skills of a high order.

Readers will also be impressed by the sensitive understanding in the presentation of the psychosocial situation of the laid-off workers: both the stresses on them and their families that inevitably accompany layoff and the resistance to seeking and accepting outside help that has been traditionally exhibited by blue-collar workers. The detailed account of the latter phenomenon, in the chapter on the Southgate project, confirms Lerner's hypothesis of widespread "self-blaming" among blue-collar American workers. The presentation of the wide range of mental and physical health problems of the laid-off Southgate workers and their families, and the methods of combating them, is both revelatory and an important original contribution.

Finally, I wish to commend organizers of these programs (and the book's authors) on their understanding and incorporation of the resource of self-help groups in furthering their objectives. Especially in dealing with immobilizing subjective reactions to life crises and disruptions, the experiences described again demonstrate that such groups, in which people affected by similar problems come together to learn coping and action skills, are an invaluable and versatile social resource.

ALFRED H. KATZ
School of Public Health
University of California, Los Angeles

Preface

This book describes the psychosocial intervention programs that were developed to assist displaced workers, a newer classification of the unemployed, in coping with the stresses associated with a major life transition. The unemployed have been viewed as a single entity, namely individuals without jobs regardless of duration, circumstance, or choice. Social and political biases have precluded making objective distinctions between the chronically or long-term unemployed and others who are situationally out of work, such as the displaced or dislocated workers. These are individuals who have been terminated or laid off due to plant closure or relocation. The stresses of job loss on these workers place them and their families at high risk for physical and emotional problems.

Current studies of stress, coping, and adaptation have provided scientific evidence linking job loss, subsequent unemployment, and occupational change with a variety of emotional and physical illnesses. Empirical research has shown statistically significant correlations between unemployment and increased first admissions to mental health facilities, suicides, homicides, imprisonment, and mortality. Despite this, displaced workers have not availed themselves of mental health services. This is particularly true of older, blue-collar workers. A specially designed approach to providing interventions to this group and other displaced workers resulted in the innovations reported upon in this book.

These prevention programs were designed to assist individuals to make important decisions regarding job change, retraining, and possible relocation, in order to reduce the traumatic effects of job loss. The book explores issues related to psychological attachment to the workplace, as well as the impact of job loss on the individual, the family, and the affected community. In addition, the book includes a review of the current literature on the health and mental health effects of job loss.

While current research has indicated the health and mental health costs of unemployment, there is a lag between this knowledge and the technical skills to provide effective interventions. Many previous attempts have been made by mental health professionals to offer assistance to those suffering job loss. These efforts, however, have had difficulty attracting participants, perhaps because of the stigma attached to them. Mental health professionals have had difficulty modifying their interventions to attract non-clinical populations who are undergoing transitional stress. Personnel managers and vocational counselors frequently have lacked the requisite clinical skills to meet the specific emotional needs of these populations. This book includes some practical tools to assist these professionals in the design and implementation of an effective counseling program.

This book will present to the reader the common reactions to job loss, problems of adaptation, and concepts of transition, as well as the more extreme and pathological responses. This information will be of use to a range of human service providers: mental health professionals, personnel managers, vocational and rehabilitation counselors, labor organizations, and manpower agency staff. Information is included that will be useful in planning and implementing effective crisis intervention programs for displaced workers, the chronically unemployed, and others affected by technological change. The crucial transitional phases contributing to unemployment stress, such as plant closure, layoff, retraining, and employment in new occupations, are discussed.

This book is a result of the hands-on experiences of the authors in working with displaced workers. The health and mental health promotion and primary prevention model has now been used with such groups as autoworkers, steelworkers, aerospace workers, cannery workers, hospital service workers, and electronic assembly workers. This innovative intervention program model has been well received by training institutions, labor unions, government employment development agencies, and, most important, those experiencing job loss. The model of intervention reported here has been designed not only to provide ready accessibility to services, but also to eliminate the stigma frequently associated with mental health services in order to encourage help-seeking.

1

Community Crisis: Individual and Collective Responses to Job Loss

ADAPTATION TO JOB LOSS

Plant closings and mass layoffs have become commonplace in the 1980s. Unemployment and displacement due to technological change have resulted in profound economic and emotional consequences for diverse populations in the United States (Bluestone & Harrison, 1982). The stresses of unemployment on displaced workers and their families increase their vulnerability to economic and emotional disruptions (Newman, 1988). Sudden job loss is a crisis event in the life of an individual. A mass layoff or plant closing becomes a collective stressor to those who share a workplace. Each person, however, develops a unique set of coping responses to these shared stressors and each constructs a framework for making sense of what happened.

Sociopsychological and sociological studies of plant closings and mass industrial layoffs have not indicated the presence of individual pathology. Displaced workers reported experiencing only limited emotional impacts in such areas as psychosocial stresses and somatic responses (Buss & Redburn, 1981; Kasl & Cobb, 1979; Little, 1976). One recent study, however, found considerable family stresses, various somatic complaints, and increased smoking and alcohol use among displaced workers (Rayman & Bluestone, 1982a, b).

Psychiatric epidemiological studies have been undertaken, as well, to document the longer-term effects of unemployment on mental health. A national probability sample of jobless men, studied over a seven-year period, indicated more feelings of powerlessness, decreased motivation, and increased physical health problems than with the control population (Parnes & King, 1977). A recent panel survey found that unemployed men experienced significantly greater depression, anxiety, and somaticism than working controls, and indicated that these symptoms increased over time with extended unemployment (Liem, Atkinson, & Liem, 1982).

Psychoeconomic studies view the problem as emerging from socioeconomic conditions. Catalano and Dooley (1977) used macroeconomic data to predict statistically mental health effects of joblessness from interview data gathered over a 16-month period. They found significant relationships among economic change, mood state, and stressful life events. Using microeconomic data and public records, Brenner (1973, 1980) found significant relationships between unemployment and admissions to psychiatric facilities. Brenner's national probability study, based upon data generated during the recession of the early 1970s, links a 14.3% increase in unemployment to a 6% rise in arrests and mental hospital admissions, a 1% increase in suicides, and a 2.3% increase in death from all types of causes.

There are few indicators of severe mental illness concomitant with job loss. Individual responses to the event, however, may vary with respect to emotional functioning and adaptive coping. Although a mass layoff is an intrusive event, most program planners and clinicians make assumptions about the help-seeking behavior of the target population. Their *a priori* judgments are often based on evidence reported in previous studies and their experiences with other populations. Most of these studies report low utilization of services by displaced workers. This pattern of help seeking may reflect their loss of health insurance benefits and a lack of information regarding public health services. A study was conducted of 1,332 unemployed individuals residing in the Detroit tricounty area regarding health insurance, use of health care services, and health status. It was found that over half of the group had no health insurance coverage when they were unemployed; 78% had coverage when they were employed; and 37% of this group had at least one chronic condition (Berki, Lichtenstein, & Wyszewianski, 1984).

When clinical interventions for the unemployed are sponsored by mental health centers, and therefore identified as mental health programs, there tends to be low utilization of services. The presumption of pathology is often used to justify these services and the resulting expenditures. Efforts to deliver conventional mental health services by those clinicians who have observed the consequences of joblessness, have been for the most part unsuccessful. When a publicly funded mental health agency in the Pacific Southwest, for example, assigned a clinical social worker to a local union hall that was affected by a recent plant closure, there was a very low utilization of her services. Most displaced workers perceive their problem to be joblessness and economic need, and this is often the case.

THE CRISIS OF JOB LOSS

When a layoff or plant closure occurs, multiple perspectives emerge: those of the displaced workers, of the union leadership, of the managers of the company, and of the providers of human services to the affected population. The emotional consequences of the crisis, however, are of greatest significance to the displaced workers. These individuals must successfully transfer technical and coping skills derived from previous life crises in order to resolve the current crisis. Job loss is a crisis of competence that challenges people to consider their sources of vulnerability and strength, and to reconstruct their lives. Individuals must be willing to confront issues of occupational choice and job satisfaction, as well as to face the necessity of maintaining a work life and a set of adult responsibilities, in order to weather this crisis successfully.

Longer-term workers face a greater challenge, that of self-efficacy. They must examine their capacity to make a life change, despite an often-held personal belief that they are too old to reenter the labor market and are not attractive to potential employers. An emergent issue for the older worker is personal competence and self-confidence in the ability to seek, and perhaps retrain for, meaningful work during middle adulthood. Older workers may perceive work differently than do their younger peers, in that they often derive a sense of personal identity and competence from their commitment to a work role, not merely to a job itself.

The work role, when viewed as a life anchor and a form of centering, enhances one's self-image as a functional, financially independent, and thereby competent adult. The stresses associated with sudden job loss may, therefore, disrupt the balance of an adult's life, and may temporarily render that person dysfunctional as well. The individual's perception, however, that she or he can mobilize inherent skills or competencies to cope effectively with this crisis may contribute to what has been called a sense of self-empowerment. The conscious sense of oneself as a fully empowered adult may be the emergent strength, or virtue, of those who can acknowledge, struggle, and successfully cope with the challenges of sudden job loss as a crisis of competence.

The crisis of job loss changes the lives of the affected individuals, as well as the institutions and communities that sustain them. The crisis is a stressful event that disrupts the balance within these macrosystems (O'Connor, 1987). Macro-level organizational strategies often develop as an adaptive response to this event (Alexander, 1987; Miller, 1978). Organizations and communities, like individuals, may have to draw upon competencies derived from adjusting to past crises. These affected systems may not previously have incurred this specific type of event. Their decision-makers must, therefore, call upon strategies that have facilitated effective institutional coping with similar critical incidents. The experience of the event itself and the emergent pattern of responses will influence the direction of change within these macrosystems through later stages of their development.

Emergent subsystems will often develop within a community's institutional life to support the affected individuals. In smaller communities, for example, there is often coalition building among health, mental health, and social service providers, and charitable organizations. In larger, urban regions, this form of community support is inhibited because of the geographic dispersal of the workers themselves. The broader geographical base of a company's work force diffuses alliances with peers, with natural or formal helpers in the union or plant, and with local service providers. The event may appear to be more encapsulated and the ripple effect less immediately evident in urban regions. The immediate effect is noticeable, although moderately, in the area contiguous to the plant itself. The event is somewhat moderated, however, by the fact that most workers reside outside of the communities in which they are employed and commute to the work site. In southern California, for example, most employees do not reside in "company towns." The newer high-technology industrial plants are often located in a recently developed industrial park area within an urban region. The workers themselves, moreover, have not become integrated into the institutional life of the communities adjacent to these industrial parks. The impact of the layoff, therefore, often goes unnoticed by neighbors, media, community leaders, and service providers. The sense of anonymity that results from this situation further isolates the individuals who are experiencing this collective stressor and who are attempting to make sense of it. Community influentials will often view the event as minimally significant to the flow of institutional life, and this perception limits their efforts to mobilize collective support on behalf of the affected population.

The crisis of job loss carries with it a sense of irony and incongruity, that of being "down and out" in an affluent society. This is often the dilemma of the worker who, at midlife and midcareer, finds that her or his skills are obsolete and, therefore, not transferable. The middle-aged worker will often deny this reality and resist efforts to upgrade skills or to change careers, even after having had up to a year's warning that a layoff might occur. The following cases point to this process of crisis, resistance, and directive change at the individual and collective levels.

CASE

A 47-year-old chemist, who was employed with a firm for 17 years in a middle-management position, was aware that his company had merged with a larger corporation and that changes would likely result from the reorganization. He chose, however, to remain with the firm until the actual layoff took place. His explanation for this decision was that he believed that, at his age, he would not be in the job market again. He had expected to remain with that firm until retirement age. When the layoff actually occurred, he blamed himself for not having aggressively sought other employment. He welcomed the several weeks of "paid vacation" that the severance pay would provide. However, he found himself unsettled and unable to enjoy his "time out." He reported that anxiety, fatigue, and depression inhibited his motivation to take the necessary steps in looking for a new job.

Other individuals are able to mobilize their resources towards job search and bring about such career changes earlier in the pre-layoff period, that is, once they know that their job will be coming to an end. These are often workers who have more job mobility because their skills are more transferable. Many of these displaced workers in the current labor market, however, have never been in this situation before, nor have they ever had to undertake a directed job-search effort. They had previously found their jobs through different strategies and during an earlier period of their lives when the labor market was far more open. This is true essentially for blue-collar, semi-skilled, or unskilled workers, many of whom have emigrated from other countries and were not able to transfer their skills to the American labor market. Many of these workers were initially attracted to companies known for providing good benefit packages to their employees or where there was a strong labor union to provide protection.

CASE

A large number of low-income, unskilled cannery workers were recently displaced from their jobs. This group comprised predominantly middle-aged women with minimal literacy and represented a variety of ethnic backgrounds, including Black, Hispanic, Asian, and Eastern European. There was an extreme sense of emotional loss as a result of this mass layoff. Their reaction was particularly striking because the work they did was tedious, repetitive, and, in general, unpleasant. The plant was damp and odoriferous, and the work done was boning and packing of large fish. The women's work stations were raised wooden platforms with 12 to 16 women at each work station. Despite this physically unpleasant work environment, morale was reported to be quite high. There was a strong sense of intimacy among these women, and within the plant in general. There were many families with several members employed in the plant, and this facilitated a sense of connectedness. There were some ethnic and national subgroupings, and reports of favoritism for promotions and exclusion from particular tasks because of these differences. Nevertheless, very few people reported dissatisfaction with their work, and many expressed sadness about the loss of the "work family."

The members of this work force faced serious problems in adapting to this collective crisis because of their lack of skill and literacy. The persistent theme encountered in their discussion of job loss was disappointment because of their expectation of permanence in the employment at the cannery. They often expressed feelings of abandonment by the company, disillusionment with the union, and increasing despair regarding new employment. The workers felt a great sense of isolation after the plant closed. It was difficult for them to visualize another work setting, separated from their peers, where they would be autonomous. In their job search, for example, they would travel together, two or three in a car, for a job interview. Most of these workers had found their jobs at the cannery through familial or social network contacts. The workplace, with its closely knit social support system or "work family," effectively kept them from either lateral movement in their occupations or full participation in the labor market. Job search was thus a particularly difficult experience for them, since many were monolingual, lived and worked in the same geographical area, and were strongly interdependent for their transportation and their social needs.

The example of the cannery workers illustrates a process of attachment, separation, and loss with respect to a workplace that was originally conceptualized by Bowlby in his works with reference to other contexts (1973, 1980, 1982). These cannery workers were long-term employees who perceived the workplace as a family or social network that protected them emotionally, as well as economically. The more strongly attached to this work family they were, the more traumatic was the separation process. Many of these workers felt a tremendous sense of abandonment and disillusionment when the layoff occurred and the plant was closed. The "myth of security" that attracted them to the plant was destroyed. They had expected to remain with the company permanently. The satisfaction with the work was of secondary importance to job security and the camaraderie within the workplace.

WORKPLACE ATTACHMENT AND JOB LOSS

Bowlby's attachment theory (Jacobson, 1987; Marris, 1982; Petrovich & Gewirtz, 1985) applies to both group-level and individual-level phenomena with respect to workplace attachment, separation, and loss. This insight arises from the belief that the workplace is a significant social system to which an individual becomes attached through affiliations with others in the setting. Common ties emerge through time spent working together and sharing a role with respect to a specific authority structure, such as relationships and perceptions of supervisors, the company, and its management. The term "work family" has frequently been attributed to this set of relationships. It is not accidental that the quasi-kin terminology of "brothers and sisters" is commonly used by union leaders to instill and reinforce relational ties among rank and file members.

Two factors appear to influence the attachment of an individual to a workplace. The first—personal attachment style— develops through the history of an individual's experience of attachment, separation, loss, and competence in the family and other contexts outside of the workplace (Bloom-Feshbach & Bloom-Feshbach, 1987; Cohler & Stott, 1987; Field, 1985; Piotrkowski & Gornick, 1987; Reite & Capitanio, 1985). The second— workplace attachment style—emerges from an individual's work history and the level, the limitations, and the transferability of job skills. Therefore, for the person who has had a lengthy relationship with one company, threatened loss creates a type of crisis and separation similar to that experienced during bereavement, divorce, and larger-scale events such as residential loss following urban relocation and disaster (Erikson, 1976; Fried, 1963; Marris, 1974; Parkes, 1982; Young & Willmott, 1957).

The paradigm of attachment theory has demonstrated value for understanding the individual's responses to processes of change. It is a useful model, too, for planning programs that address both intrapsychic and sociopsychological issues associated with sudden job loss. The following description of stages of job loss and separation from the workplace demonstrates how this model can be a viable framework for planning clinical and social interventions for displaced workers.

Stage 1: Preparatory Efforts

In most job situations, the usual practice had been to notify the employee two to four weeks before termination. Under the current federal Economic Dislocation and Worker Adjustment Assistance Act, when a plant closure or layoff affects 50 or more employees, the company is required to provide 60 days notice. This federal legislation mandates shared participation of work-

ers, management and labor organizatinos and specifies the
state's responsibility for the utilization and allocatin of federal
funds. Basic mandated services include the development of
an individual readjustment plan for participants, retraining services and supportive services, including vocational and personal counseling.

In unionized workplaces, management notifies the union of
the pending reduction in the work force. Management and
union officials negotiate issues of seniority, benefits, severance
pay, and the timetable for the layoff or closure. Information
regarding these projected actions flows through both formal
and informal networks. Media reports on economic issues,
such as production flows, mergers, and cutbacks in the industry, usually precede and accompany this process. Many
employees may begin to seek work elsewhere. Older workers
and others who have been with the company for a longer time
have a longer-term investment, and are often reluctant to take
action during this preliminary stage. In larger companies, for
example, there are benefits that will accrue to these longer-
term workers at layoff, such as early retirement and severance
pay. These considerations, however, may have both negative
and positive implications for the employee and will often affect an individual's motivations and willingness to seek occupational change.

Stage 2: First Responses to the Event

Leaders of progressive labor unions appear to have a more
enlightened level of awareness and understanding of job loss.
The emotional significance of this economic crisis has become
commonly acknowledged. Unions have had increased awareness of drug and alcohol problems at the work site. Union-
sponsored substance abuse treatment programs have been provided to their members by on-site counselors as well as
industry-based employee assistance plans. Union benefit
packages often include mental health coverage. Workers

themselves are becoming more familiar with counseling services to assist them with family problems and stresses. Increasing numbers of larger companies are subscribing to prepaid mental health plans. Larger unions, such as the United Auto Workers, have been at the forefront in providing mental health services to their members through their early involvement with community mental health centers. This has also been true of such unions as the Retail Clerks, which at one time operated its own mental health clinics. The AFL-CIO Federation has sponsored training programs for shop stewards as work-site intervenors for drug and alcohol problems. The Institute for Labor and Mental Health in Oakland has also provided training programs for shop stewards from several major unions in the San Francisco Bay area who deal with the mental health problems of workers through the creation of occupational stress groups.

Union leaders have shown a strong sense of responsibility for the workers facing layoff. The unions themselves have decreasing power, however, in affecting the decisions leading to plant closures and mass layoffs. These labor organizations, then, are themselves in crisis since they are unable to protect their members from job loss. There are increasingly strong anti-union sentiments among workers in general, and particularly during a crisis period, such as prior to a mass layoff. Workers frequently blame the union for their job loss.

It is frequently the union leaders who experience the anger, frustration, and despair of the rank-and-file members, who seek assistance for their constituency. Their motives are often self-protective since they feel inadequate to respond both personally and on behalf of their organization to their members' needs. They fear such catastrophic consequences as suicide and serious psychosomatic reactions. The term "stress" is frequently used, rather than psychological or mental disorder, to describe the circumstances of their membership. Under ordinary working conditions, the shop steward and committee member can utilize peer support systems, on-site substance abuse counselors, or mental health resources. When the layoff occurs, however, this support structure for the worker is gone. Insurance benefits end at layoff or extend for a circumscribed period of time. With some exceptions, the retirement-aged worker may have lifetime health insurance coverage. In anticipation of the impending situation, the more enlightened union leaders become concerned about the repercussions of their members' anger and disillusionment. Many companies acknowledge these same problems in their work force as layoff approaches, and hire out-placement firms to assist in resume writing and job-search workshops. In some rare instances, these companies also offer stress-reduction or other workshops, usually targeted to middle management.

Stage 3: The Call for Help

Union leaders, personnel managers, and members of the occupational health team often feel isolated as they observe changes in the atmosphere of the workplace as their co-workers become distressed during this pre-layoff period. Many of the workers approach these influentials to voice concerns regarding the layoff and its implications for the course of their lives. Very often, clear information is lacking regarding such issues as the dates of termination or severance pay. This renders these natural helpers essentially ineffective in offering their assistance. Once the decision has been made from the "top down" to close a plant or reduce the work force the union and middle management have lost their constituency, namely, the rank-and-file workers for whom they have served as negotiator and advocate. They are often threatened with termination themselves.

Sometimes a member of the human services system will initiate the call for help. Members of action-oriented labor unions will often initiate spontaneous, voluntary self-help efforts, such as food banks, holiday toy campaigns, and outreach within the labor movement. The union hall is a supportive environment during this stage and its space is "reenergized" with new tasks and roles, and the sudden acknowledgment that "we are on our own." New leadership emerges to serve a constituency that is facing an impending crisis, one that the departing leadership is unprepared to manage. There are many questions, for example, raised by rank-and-file members regarding their immediate needs as well as future needs.

Troubled workers who are facing a layoff or plant closure often delay seeking help from outside agencies because of feelings of confusion about what is taking place. There is an initial sense of disbelief and denial. The work situation often places the group of employees in a tightly bound network of relationships. Their work life and, to a certain extent, their social life are spatially and temporally organized around a routine of shift work and car pools, that require fixed behavioral repertoires. These individuals are therefore facing, along with the loss of their jobs, the loss of a pattern of living, marked by changed cyclical rhythms of waking and sleeping, eating and socializing. The external threat of the impending layoff or plant closure encapsulates the workers from the community, and frequently from their families. It is not unusual for a worker to withhold information about the pending layoff from family members and friends. Some workers have tried to conceal this information after they have been laid off by leaving the house each morning and returning home at the end of the day. Union leaders and corporate management often attempt to mask or deny the reality by conducting "business as usual" up to the closing date. Delay, masking, and denial effectively serve to shelter an individual from acknowledging that she or he has a problem and may need help. This is not to imply a flagrant display of psychiatric symptomatology. These defense mechanisms are, rather, signs that an individual is attempting to minimize the crisis. They are the key areas of concern in a program of early intervention and primary prevention of stress reactions during layoff or plant closure.

In larger-scale layoffs, where a wider spectrum of workers is affected, reports begin to circulate regarding the fate of those who have already lost their jobs. These reports include suicide attempts, heart attacks, family breakdown, and very often excessive drinking and drug use. Early reports of severe economic problems, such as default on mortgages, are circulated as well.

The critical incident, however, that inspires help seeking is often an actual personal tragedy.

Stage 4: Disillusionment

During this stage, displaced workers often express a need for detachment from the process of change. They are disillusioned and are afraid to let go of their work-like routines. They attempt to camouflage this fear of letting go as a way of protecting the ego from the pain that arises from confronting change. The outward signs of this letting go manifest as focused anger, denial, attribution of blame to others, and the early signs of self-blame. One of the first manifestations of impending job loss is anger, often resulting from frustration and attribution of blame directed towards the employer, the union, and such general conditions as foreign competition and lower worker-performance standards. The less competent the individual in terms of limited job skills and job experiences, the more detached that person appears to be from the process of change. For example, a worker who has been employed in a job with a singular task is at a greater disadvantage economically because she or he has fully adapted to this type of work role on a socio-psychological level. Further research is necessary, however, on the relationship between minimal work skills and psychological adaptation, including the capacity for change.

With more competent workers—that is, those who have acquired a repertoire of multiple skills in a variety of work settings—the focus of attention shifts to the coping process necessary for successful transition. Coping skills needed during this transition are self-esteem, awareness of options, a sense of direction, and following through on job-search strategies. These individuals are better able to mobilize systems that provide support for change.

With less competent workers, this detachment from the change process becomes self-defeating. They often direct their energies in their final weeks at the old workplace to fighting issues of termination, rather than to considering their options and seeking work elsewhere. These workers continue to believe that the present job will continue and accuse the union of not "fighting" for their interests. These expressions of power-lessness appear in a variety of ways. Some individuals make extreme statements of helplessness and "devotion." Frequently heard, as well, are statements of loyalty to the company from individuals of all skill levels—from nurse's aides and assembly workers to administrative personnel. Others express their perceived importance to the labor process in their workplace and lament the lack of appreciation by the company for their years of commitment. What is striking is how little the nature of the work relates to an individual's reaction to job loss. Employees at every level express concern about the company's termination policies regarding severance pay, health insurance and unemployment benefits, and the actual date of layoff. It is difficult for them to engage in more constructive efforts at this stage.

One of the trouble signs of this stage is the anxious attach-ment to the job and the workplace. The work often does not provide the individual with gratification, achievement motiva-tion, or inherent job satisfaction. The sole gratification is the paycheck received at the end of the week. Many jobs lack skill transferability. For some people, it is the awareness of what they have been doing day by day for so many years that brings about a sense of disillusionment. In the past, those in an organized workplace perceived management and the company as a common adversary. When a closure is about to take place, the disillusionment with the union begins to occur, cutting through the "we–they" dichotomy that underlies the discourse of union members. But this serves only to increase their sense of powerlessness because the workers' identification with the union and any perceived solidarity with peers are breaking down.

What is very striking during this period of termination is how few of these workers seek other job possibilities. In organized workplaces, they are inhibited by questions of possi-

ble work recall and severance pay that may be under negotiation. The workers are often insecure about making an early
job change because of the economic issues created by the labor
contracts and their future unemployment insurance benefits.
Since their sense of job security, as well as their confidence,
has been undermined by the impending job loss, they are fear-
ful that the new job will offer no security. There is ambivalence
about the future. The recently purchased home, recreational
vehicle, and other symbols of upward mobility reflect their
plans for the future. The dreams of retirement fostered by
longevity in a workplace are now being shattered. It appears
that individuals who cope better with this forced change are
those with more diversified work experience and more interests
outside the workplace that complement their jobs. There seems
to be a greater sense of optimism among these workers, and
they tend to perceive the process of change as an opportunity.

Stage 5: Acceptance

This stage is marked by the individual's acknowledgment
of the need for action and the inevitability of change. It can
be compared to the acceptance of loss described by Kubler-
Ross (1969) and Bowlby (1980) and the conceptual framework
of bereavement. This acceptance is often provisional, as workers
perceive the economic necessity in their situation and are skeptical about their prospects in the labor market. Recurrent
themes such as "There are no jobs out there" and "Who is going to hire me?" are openly voiced by older workers, disabled
workers, and some lesser skilled women. This stage carries
within it a sense of hesitation and overt anxiety over the impending forced change. It is not unusual for people to continue to express their anger along with the acceptance of their
crisis.
    During this stage, there is often a surge of energy as workers
begin to look for jobs and seek retraining programs. Representatives from a variety of agencies—including the state employment department, and educational, training, and mental health

service providers—introduce themselves to the displaced worker. The person becomes action-oriented and goal-oriented, which may be the sign of resilience and emotional health. The person who is seeking emancipation from the "work family" often pulls away from the union and the company. This is not to imply that there has been a strong attachment to the union or the employer. For many, it was strictly an opportunistic attachment for the purpose of economic benefit rather than of ideology.

The attributes of personal competence and self-confidence are the emergent strengths that individuals possess after successfully coping with their crisis. This acceptance stage marks a falling-away period for those who are less competent and have lower self-esteem and self-confidence. From an objective point of view, these people can vary along this dimension of competence. Job skill is not the sole variable to be considered in predicting a successful transition to new employment. Rather, success is the result of a combination of external criteria, such as job skills, work history, and psychological strengths. Many individuals lack internal strengths to cope with the crisis of job loss and have greater difficulty moving into this stage. From a theoretical point of view, it appears that a maladaptive attachment process occurs between workers and the workplace during their years of employment in that setting. This often stems from the loss of empowerment emerging from the dehumanization of the work routine and the fear of loss of jobs, particularly those that require low skills and rote tasks and therefore little exploration. These jobs also lack the conditions and incentives for personal growth, such as job variety and job satisfaction, and serve to limit the worker's sense of self-esteem and personal competence. Many look upon job change from a strictly economic viewpoint. The expression "We can always get another job" is often heard from those who have changed jobs frequently because of industry conditions or burnout caused by boredom or rage over the work situation. Such job changes are often lateral. It appears less difficult for these workers to accept the need for change because their attachment to the present job and the workplace is more superficial and tentative, which creates greater ease in mobility. Among the lesser skilled workers, the job is not endowed with aspirations to career and social status. Although this superficial attachment is more characteristic of people with limited educational level and lower socioeconomic status, it has been observed as well among the most highly skilled workers in "demand" occupations in the labor market. Until recently, this was particularly true of those employed in the computer and other high-technology fields, where the influx of venture capital provided opportunities for rapid career growth and advancement in newly formed enterprises.

For workers who have either self-imposed or realistically grounded geographical limitations, this stage of acceptance brings with it a deep sense of despair. They see few options available in the proximate locality and are unable to envision themselves moving to a new community for employment. There have been major migrations for purposes of seeking work throughout this century. Southern Black and Appalachian White workers "went north" to find work in the industrial Midwest; and there were migrations from the southwestern "Dustbowl" states to find work in the fields and canneries of California during the Great Depression. More recently, there have been migrations to the "Sunbelt" states to seek jobs in the high-technology fields of aerospace and electronics. Currently, such economic opportunities do not appear to exist for the less-skilled workers. They seem to be more uncomfortable with leaving a familiar environment for an uncertain future. The prospect of separation from residential and community ties, combined with the crisis of job loss, places the newly unemployed at greater risk of emotional and socioeconomic maladaptation.

The community-crisis paradigm, therefore, reflects the individual's search for stability and balance in view of the uncertainty of an unstable collective event. Job loss as part of a plant closing or mass industrial layoff is conceptualized as a collective stressor. The sense of consistency between the individual and the collectivity derives from a person's ability to cope with the crisis by using the institutional resources available within the community. The crisis intervention model that has been useful in such areas as disaster, urban relocation, bereavement, chronic illness, and disability is also applicable when job loss occurs, because it identifies (1) the stages of the crisis; (2) the hazard to the individual; and (3) individual strengths, including personal coping strategies.

2

The Mental Health of Displaced Workers: An Overview

In the light of our present awareness of the relationship between the problems of unemployment and mental health and psychiatric conditions, it is hard to imagine that only a decade ago our attitudes were very different (Liem, 1987). In the past, unemployment was considered from the point of view of economics and essentially as a reflection of the business cycle. It was also seen as a consequence of mental illness rather than as a cause. The first systematic, sociological studies of job loss and unemployment and their effects on individuals, families, and communities appeared in the 1930s during the world depression. These studies focused on the relationship of unemployment and poverty and as a source of social instability (Bakke, 1940; Eisenberg & Lazarsfeld, 1938; Jahoda, Lazarsfeld, & Zeisel, 1971). In the 1960s, when the U. S. community mental health center movement evolved, attention was still predominantly given to the economic aspects of unemployment, with the focus mostly on minorities who were victims of racial discrimination. In the 1970s and 1980s researchers have begun to explore the effects of unemployment on the health and mental health of the community and its members. Community mental health centers have themselves played only a relatively minor role in addressing this individual, family, community, and social problem, and, despite the disruption of entire communities, have developed few programs to meet the mental health needs of displaced workers. This is explained in part by the centers' diminishing resources, which must be devoted to the chronically mentally ill and the homeless.

An early, wide-ranging review article by Eisenberg and Lazarsfeld (1938) of 100 studies of unemployment during the depression years found relatively little mention of anxiety and depression. The study by Jahoda, Lazarsfeld, and Zeisel (1971) of the closing of a textile mill in Marienthal, Austria, was notable for its detailed description of social conditions and reactions and of the distinct stages in the response to forced unemployment: initial shock, followed by optimism, then pessimism and anxiety, and finally, fatalism or resignation. A study by Bakke (1940) of workers and families in England and the United States only noted that physical and mental exhaustion appeared in the worker and family when the search for a job was unsuccessful. Liem (1987) concluded that the authors of these two studies saw the results of unemployment as stages of adaptation and accommodation to severely diminished economic opportunities.

Liem's (1987) review of the studies of unemployment during the depression years of the 1930s noted a significant difference between the conditions of that early depression and the more recent recessions of today. The early depression produced massive unemployment and severe economic losses, while the recessions of today have been accompanied by more modest levels of unemployment. Job loss has been experienced more as a private problem. Liem concludes that the changes are the results of today's conditions providing a number of social safety nets to some workers, better standards of living, a more highly educated work force, greater participation by women in the labor force, and a much more involved public service sector.

TYPES OF RESEARCH

In their review of the literature, Buss and Redburn (1983) classified the studies of unemployment into three groups: case studies of the unemployed and profiles of their families and/or communities experiencing massive job losses and economic hardships (Bakke, 1940; Jahoda, 1979; Jahoda, Lazarsfeld, & Zeisel, 1971; Komarovsky, 1940); empirical studies relating job loss and unemployment to social disorders and individual mental dysfunction (Brenner, 1973, 1976; Catalano & Dooley, 1977); and cross-sectional statistical analyses of the relationship between measures of unemployment or employment status and selected indicators of social and psychological status (Caplovitz, 1979; Dohrenwend & Dohrenwend, 1974; Durman, 1976).

In the authors' opinion, the case study approach has been valuable in providing an understanding of the dynamics involved in human response to economic stresses; the aggregate approach has been rewarding with increasingly sophisticated studies that examined the relationship between economic change, social stress, and emotional disorders; and the cross-sectional analyses have thus far revealed relatively little about the dynamics of disorder development or whether economic hardship is the cause or the result of emotional disorder.

A highly selective review of the literature on the emotional stress of unemployment, the physical reactions, and the current view of social supports as buffers follows. This chapter will also describe a few of the varied programs developed by community mental health and other resources of the community in response to unemployment and job loss.

EMOTIONAL STRESS/DISTRESS IN JOB LOSS AND UNEMPLOYMENT

A methodology for analyzing mental health effects of unemployment emerged in the 70s from the development of a stress paradigm in the social and behavioral sciences (Liem, 1987). Within this paradigm, unemployment was transformed into a social stressor, allowing psychological analysis. Unemployment was found to be one of the best predictors of emotional strain, with job loss and demotion to be two of the strongest predictors of depression (Perlin & Lieberman, 1979). Cobb and Kasl's (1977) early study of groups of individuals who were followed through the experience of job loss and the subsequent period of unemployment after plant closings is an excellent example of the case study approach. Despite a small sample size, the results were important because the study design included measurements made prior to plant closings and accompanying layoffs. The information was gathered over a two-and-a-half-year period and included health readings, questionnaire measures of mental health, and data on changes in economic circumstances. Control data were collected from workers in plants not threatened with closure. The researchers concluded that the experience of job loss was stressful, requiring at least several months for the person to return to normal, and was associated with such psychological symptoms as increased depression, anomie, anger/irritation, and suspicion. Job loss also produced a rise in risk factors for physical health, such as coronary heart disease, along with other health problems, like dyspepsia, joint swelling, hypertension, and alopecia. Suicide risk was also increased. Cobb and Kasl stressed that their statistical measures did not fully capture the degree of anguish experienced by workers and their families.

An early aggregate study by Brenner (1973) did much to stimulate research on the psychological effects of unemployment. In his study, Brenner examined indicators of economic change in relation to institutional measures of psychological impairment. He analyzed the relationship between annual rates of employment and psychiatric hospital admissions for New York State for a period from 1850 to 1967. Brenner found that admissions followed downturns in the economy by two or three years for many groups of psychiatric patients. Subsequent studies by Brenner reported similar findings for other localities in both the United States and Europe.

The relationship between psychiatric inpatient and outpatient admissions over a 100-month period (1971 to 1979) and monthly state unemployment percentages for the same period was investigated in Missouri by Ahr, Gorodezky, and Cho

(1981). The overall data did not show any significant relationship between first admissions for the total population and unemployment. However, when special subpopulations were identified, significant correlations emerged. Thus, the impact of unemployment for former mental patients was immediate, whereas for patients previously served by non-mental health facilities the impact was felt only after one month. Another subset, patients who were unemployed at the time of admission, was characterized by economic stress and a higher admission rate in correlation with the unemployment index than was the total patient group. In general, the findings demonstrated the importance of readmissions to mental health facilities in relation to unemployment.

Brenner's work led to additional studies by other researchers, some of which refined Brenner's early conclusions, especially in identifying factors that might affect the results, such as shifting patterns of patient care in the community. Catalano and Dooley (1979), for example, found that a rise in psychiatric admissions during periods of rising unemployment occurred only for middle class samples in large metropolitan areas. Therefore, treatment data for lower-class persons would not necessarily reflect recent elevations in psychological symptoms because of their traditionally lower utilization pattern.

Following Brenner's research, a number of studies on the psychological effects of unemployment came from scientists studying stressful life events, a strategy that emphasizes the cumulative stress of many events rather than the impact of a singular experience. The investigators found that economic events, especially unemployment, were among the best predictors of emotional strain. These findings were at first serendipitous and served to strengthen the connection between unemployment and psychological well-being (Holmes & Rahe, 1967; Weiner, 1974).

The situation of job loss and unemployment has been described by Kelvin and Jarrett (1985) as profoundly deindividualizing as one becomes labeled "unemployed." They report that feelings of injury and fury at dismissal or guilt with self-blame arise at plant closings, even though the event is one over which the individual has no control. The effects appear to be more marked in men than in women. Families are affected by the man's loss of self-confidence as unemployment continues, with the individual frequently feeling himself in a position of reduced authority. The man may feel the directions of dependency beginning to change, with resultant increasing strain on the marital relationship. Among friends, and especially in society, the unemployed may feel stigmatized and uneasy. Psychologically, as well as economically, unemployment is felt as a condition of forced dependence and as an assault against one's sense of "occupational identity."

A number of studies focusing on emotional reactions (Atkinson, Liem & Liem, 1986; Kasl & Cobb, 1982; Kessler, House, & Turner, 1987; Rayman & Bluestone, 1982b; Warr, 1984) found that psychological distress involved primarily depression and anxiety, with increased anger and hostility in male workers, milder precursors of discouragement, lowered esteem and self-confidence, and considerable worry. The immediate worries centered on the loss of financial resources, the loss of health insurance, and difficulties in providing for the needs of one's children. Later tensions in family relationships, the frustrations of looking for work, and anxiety about future job markets contributed to the emotional burden. Longitudinal studies indicated that depression, anxiety, and worrying generally decreased dramatically following reemployment. The anxiety and depression seemed, therefore, most accurately considered reactive and situational.

The severity of the depression and anxiety in the early stages can be high. In comparing the percentage of employed and unemployed workers scoring above the cutoff on his measure of distress, the General Health Questionnaire, Warr (1984) found 54% to 62% of the unemployed scoring above the cutoff compared with 15% to 25% among the employed used as controls. Cobb and Kasl (1977) and Kasl and Cobb (1979), in their follow-up studies of plant closings, found that the greatest insecurity about the future and highest feelings of job deprivation occurred shortly before the actual layoffs for blue-collar workers. Some relief was experienced at the time of the closings, followed by inconsistent fluctuations in distress over the two-year study period.

The pattern of depression was even more unpredictable. Kasl and Cobb (1979) concluded that the assumption of harmful longer-term psychological effects of unemployment was not warranted empirically. Liem (1987), however, points out that these studies were done during a period of general economic growth rather than decline and that this may have accounted for some of the variability in the results. Liem concluded that when jobs were available, chronic and characterological depression was probably one of the factors contributing to a worker's inability or lack of desire to return to work.

Liem's (1983) study of workers in the aerospace industry showed increased headaches, gastrointestinal distress, and elevated blood pressure, along with heightened anxiety and worry, increased drinking and smoking, and generalized fatigue and lethargy in those who were unemployed. The difficulties were especially pronounced among middle-aged heads of households with young dependents and among workers with at least six months of unemployment. According to this study, women who were laid off experienced greater psychological stress than men.

Depression, anxiety, hostility, suspiciousness, and somatic complaints were much more common in a group of people who had lost their jobs than in their employed counterparts (Liem, 1987). The difficulties appeared shortly after job loss, worsened over the next several months, stabilized during midyear, and then increased dramatically if unemployment continued for a year or more. Joblessness was generally more stressful for blue-collar workers than for white-collar workers. Both groups were also significantly more stressed than employed workers. Workers who blamed themselves for their job loss and failure to find new work suffered more from their unemployment than people who were able to recognize that the failing economy played a role in their fate. In general, this research has helped to negate the simplistic view that people who are depressed and anxious are not as good job hunters as less stressed persons and thus remain out of work for a longer period of time.

Liem (1987) also emphasized that a job involves more than just economics. Some workers, blue and white collars alike, find in their jobs and work sites a network of friendship and social involvement. For them the actual work is a source of personal satisfaction and achievement. These kinds of attachments to work are associated with high degrees of psychological distress during the first several months of job loss and unemployment, regardless of the financial losses that are sustained. Liem (1987) states: "The stress of employment is in part an indicator of the quality of the worker's experience on the job and the extent to which they look to paid labor as a source of personal gratification beyond economic gain" (p. 332).

Other significant factors in the worker's reaction to unemployment involve the internalization of blame for losing one's job and the duration of unemployment. In his Work and Unemployment Project, Liem (1987) found sharp rises in depression and anxiety as unemployment approached a year's duration. The pattern was different for blue- and white-collar workers. Blue-collar workers experienced an immediate rise in symptoms with more stability over time. Among white-collar workers, there was a moderate correlation between the duration of unemployment and the symptoms of distress.

Joblessness has an effect on those other than the unemployed worker. Liem (1987) found that the families of both blue- and white-collar workers showed emotional strain between husbands and wives, even when the wife also worked. The effects of unemployment on the family extended to the quality of the marital relationship and the general quality of home life. Separations and divorces occurred more often in the unemployed family. The husband's emotional state rather than the wife's reaction to the unemployment was the more important source of tension in the marriage. The strained marital relationship contributed to a decline in the cohesiveness and organization of the family as a whole. This, in turn, became a secondary source of stress for the worker and spouse.

Joelson and Whalquist (1987) described the psychological meaning of job insecurity and job loss for a group of 26 former shipyard workers and their families in Stockholm. They followed these families in depth twice a year over a two-year period and noted particularly the phases of the joblessness, the impact on identity, and the problems in adapting to a new life situation. Unemployment, especially for those over the age of 55, meant a loss of important identity-forming factors, with work as proof of one's competence and knowledge as well as a structure of relationships. Problems were especially difficult in terms of ethics, morality, and culture. They all continued to regard themselves as shipyard workers rather than as unemployed or pensioners.

The relationship between work and general psychological and physical well-being was explored by Coburn (1978) in samples of unemployed from Victoria, B. C., and families in Portland, Ore. Looking at such factors as job control, job tasks, paid job security, and bureaucratic nature of the work organization, Coburn reported that men who found their work interesting and challenging showed greater job satisfaction, even though there might be some level of associated stress. Four facets of the job stood out as having most influence on job satisfaction and feelings of alienation: prestige, control, variety, and opportunity for promotion. Pay and job security seemed unrelated.

PHASES OF REACTION TO JOB LOSS/UNEMPLOYMENT

A number of investigators have described the phases of worker reaction to job loss (Bakke, 1940; Eisenberg & Lazarsfeld, 1938; Powell & Driscoll, 1973; Root, 1979; Sloate, 1969; Taber, Walsh, & Cooke, 1979). King (1982) summarizes these findings: the initial response to rumors of termination is typically denial or disbelief; as the rumors circulate and layoffs begin, considerable anxiety mounts, especially after the first official announcement; the immediate period after termination is generally a period of relaxation, relief, and optimism, along with vigorous efforts to find a new job and with friends and family giving maximum social support; workers still unemployed four or more months after termination go through a period of vacillation and doubt, experiencing panic, rage, self-doubt, deep and potentially suicidal depression, erratic behavior, and interpersonal or marital problems; and finally, there is a period of "malaise and cynicism" in which the mood stabilizes but apathy, listlessness, resignation, and fatalism increase.

The likelihood that a given individual will experience all of these stages depends on the duration of unemployment, differences in personality, and circumstances influencing the timing and intensity of the effects.

INFLUENCE OF AGE

In general, unemployment has a more severe impact on the older worker than on the younger (Haber, Fermen, & Hudson, 1963; Kasl, Gore, & Cobb, 1975). Older workers tend to have less formal education, and the education or training they do possess often is not so relevant to their prospects for reemployment as are the skills that they acquired through work experience. Nevertheless, specialized skills of older workers are sometimes less transferable to other work settings or industries than the educational credentials of younger workers.

Frese and Mohr (1987) and Frese (1987) report a study conducted on the effects of long-term unemployment on older blue-collar workers in the Federal Republic of Germany. These researchers attempted to answer the question of whether unemployment leads to psychological depression or whether it is depressed people who are inactive and pessimistic and who will be unemployed longer. They studied unemployed blue-collar male workers in West Berlin over a period of two years, distinguishing four groups: the reemployed; unemployed throughout the entire time; reunemployed who worked in the meantime but lost jobs again; and subjects who had retired by the time of the second measurement. The authors concluded that the impact of unemployment on depression was strong and consistent.

Variables such as internal/external control, general activity levels, sickness, and age did not explain all of the effect of long-term unemployment on depression. The two unemployed groups reported decreased hope for control, increased financial problems, and increased depression. The retired and reemployed groups showed decreasing levels of financial problems and depression over time. Apparently, long-term unemployment had an impact on depression over and above the depression that occurred immediately after losing a job.

A study by Banks and Jackson (1982) focused on youth and the relationship of minor psychiatric disorders to unemployment. Their subjects consisted of two groups of young persons in England: the first, 16-year-olds interviewed at home on three occasions after leaving school; and the second, 16-year-olds interviewed at school before leaving and then twice after leaving, over approximately a year and nine months. For the first group, the second interview was about a year later and the third about one-and-a-half years after that. The results consistently indicated that the young persons who left school and continued to be unemployed showed an elevated probability of suffering from minor psychiatric disorders. The data also indicated that the experience of unemployment was more likely to create increased symptoms rather than the other way around. When the youngsters were tested while still in school, there was no difference in the psychological adjustment level. For those who left school and found work, the level of minor psychiatric disorders decreased significantly, indicating that finding employment had a protective influence. For those who experienced continued unemployment after leaving school, the mean scores increased significantly and remained at a higher level during the time they remained unemployed. When these young people became employed, the psychological disturbance score fell.

MENTAL HEALTH AND LONG-TERM UNEMPLOYMENT

Warr and Jackson (1987) investigated changes in mental health associated with enduring unemployment. The authors looked at general health, money problems, employment commitment, and social relationships among unemployed Englishmen over a period of 19 months. Interviews were at time of job loss, nine months later, and an additional 10 months after that. The results showed no change in general health or financial difficulties between the nine-month and the 19-month time period. Nevertheless, indications of general health distress remained high, well above levels in comparable employed samples.

Adaptation to unemployment was affected negatively by a strong commitment to having a job and to membership in the median age group. Such factors as availability of money, income reduction since job loss, number of dependent children, and reported financial support played no significant role. It may be that in long-term unemployment, financial routines and constraints become stabilized and constant in their effect. It was surprising to find the apparent unimportance of emotional support in relation to the adaptation to the unemployed role. The presence of a chronic health impairment did significantly reduce psychological adaptation. "Resigned adaptation" to unemployment was characterized by an impairment to aspiration, autonomy, and confidence, although the level of affective well-being was slightly higher than in the period immediately after job loss. It is worth noting that England has had high levels of unemployment for the past 20 years, with an entire generation of young persons unemployed.

Kasl and Cobb (1982) showed in a longitudinal study of plant closings and job loss how complex the situation and its measurements actually are. Job loss caused by plant closure occurred in two different companies permanently displacing their employees. One was a paint manufacturing concern in a large metropolitan area and the other a manufacturer of display fixtures in a rural community. Continuously employed men in comparable jobs in other companies were used as controls. Measurements were obtained through the various stages such as anticipation, plant closing and termination, unemployment, probationary reemployment, and stable unemployment.

The findings indicated that the men did not blame themselves for their unemployment until it continued beyond six months. Significant differences appeared in terms of both economic and work-role deprivation. Indicators of mental health status, such as depression, anxiety, and tension, showed no significant differences. Health status measures, such as complaints and disabilities, fluctuated over time but were not linked to unemployment status changes. Kasl and Cobb found evidence of adaptation in that, following the initial period of unemployment, those remaining unemployed could not be distinguished from those finding new jobs.

The investigators reported a differential effect of job loss in terms of setting, with the plant closing in the rural setting having much less significant impact than in the urban setting. Apparently, the plant closing in the rural area did not destroy the social community of co-workers, which is probably the result of a greater possibility for sharing the experience and enjoying mutual support. The investigators found that higher levels of perceived social support were associated with a lessening of the impact of the experience both physiologically and psychologically.

Persons low in social support benefited from reemployment during the early stages of job loss. In the later stages, the inadequate support appeared to increase mental health costs. The presence of psychological defenses put a person at greater risk for longer unemployment but at the same time buffered against experiencing greater job stress normally associated with the longer unemployment. Thus, psychological defenses appeared both to aggravate the exposure to an environmental stressor and to buffer its impact.

SUICIDE AND UNEMPLOYMENT

Shepherd and Barraclough (1980) reviewed a number of studies of the relationship between work and suicide, including Durkheim (1952), Sainsbury (1955), Powell (1958), Breed (1963), Sanborn, Sanborn, and Cimbolic (1974), and Morris, Kovacs, Beck and Wolffe (1974). All of the articles indicated a relationship between occupational role and suicide and that the greatest strain derived from the lack of occupation.

In their own study of 75 consecutive suicides in England, matched against a comparison group, Shepherd and Barraclough (1980) found that suicides were significantly fewer among those in full-time paid employment at the time of their death and more among those who were sick or unemployed. There was more absenteeism as a result of illness, predominantly psychiatric illness. There seemed to be more job instability, measured by number of jobs held and length of time employed. Suicides were proportionately more than twice as likely to have a high-risk occupation.

The authors concluded that the comparatively poor work record of the suicides was due to their high level of psychiatric morbidity. Work loss weakened the subject's social integration, deprived the subject of social role and status, and increased isolation, all of which contributed to despair and suicide. The authors summarized that work loss resulted from broad social and economic trends in which the unemployed's psychiatric morbidity interfered with the capacity to work, resulting in work loss with its accompanying disadvantages. Mental illness stimulated suicidal thinking and at the same time took away an effective protection against suicidal behavior.

Boor (1980) examined the suicide rates and the percentages of unemployed in the civilian labor force in eight industrial countries scattered throughout the world from 1962 to 1978 for which both unemployment rates and suicide rates were available. He found that annual variations in the suicide rates were associated positively and significantly with concomitant annual variations in the unemployment rates of six of the eight countries. Sex showed no variations in the rates, but age showed marked annual variations. For relatively young persons, increases in the suicide rates were related significantly to the increasing unemployment rates. However, the increase in unemployment rates was not related to the stable or decreasing suicide rates of older persons. Boor concluded that the social and psychological conditions in a variety of cultures that were associated with relatively high unemployment were also associated with relatively high suicide rates, especially among younger persons.

UNEMPLOYMENT AND ALCOHOL

Ames and Janes (1987b) examined the role of alcoholism in a blue-collar population and its relationship to the workplace and to unemployment. The sample was drawn from a large manufacturing plant that closed in 1982 and consisted of 30 families, 15 in which the father was a heavy drinker and 15 in which the father was a moderate drinker. After unemployment began, five of the heavy drinkers reduced their consumption to moderate levels.

Alcohol played a central role in the conduct of both work tasks and work-related leisure activities. Heavy drinkers drank on the job, during lunch breaks, and after work in parking lots, nearby bars, and selected homes where drinking was tolerated by the wives. Many who worked nights began their drinking in car pools on the way to work. Alcohol was brought into the plant in lunch boxes or thermos jugs, or stored in liquor lockers. Outside of the plant, beer was the beverage of choice; inside the plant, liquor was used because it was easier to disguise.

The reasons for excessive drinking were reported to be frequent mandatory overtime, too much free time because of the increase in mechanization, few opportunities for significant advancement (which was made largely on the basis of seniority), and high wages with exceptional benefits.

The social organization of the workplace reinforced high levels of alcohol abuse. The important factors were job alienation, job stress, inconsistent social controls, and evolution of a heavy-drinking culture. Additional characteristics were a friendship network made up mostly of fellow workers, a large proportion of leisure time spent in predominantly male peer groups, and a majority of leisure activities centered on or related to work and/or work-related social activities. Moderate drinkers, on the other hand, reported past or present involvement in religions that prohibited drinking. Their non-work social activities involved their families.

PHYSICAL HEALTH AND JOB LOSS

Cobb (1974) found that anticipation of job loss followed by the experience of unemployment resulted in elevated levels of urinary norepinephrine, creatinine, uric acid, and urea nitrogen. Norepinephrine was significantly higher prior to plant closing and persisted for 12 months afterward before it gradually lowered. Kasl and Cobb (1982) found mean diastolic and systolic blood pressure levels higher in the unemployed than in control groups.

Kessler, House, and Turner (1987) studied the effects of unemployment on health in three groups of workers: currently unemployed, previously unemployed, and stably employed. The sample was obtained through a survey of households in southeastern Michigan. Results were obtained on eight health outcomes: alcohol consumption, tranquilizer use, self-evaluated physical ill health, days restricted to bed by health problems in the last month, somatic symptoms of distress, symptoms of anxious mood, symptoms of depressed mood, and suicide thoughts in the past five years.

The results showed that the gross effects of unemployment were consistently significant, and that unemployment had a significant negative effect on all the factors except three—amount drunk, use of tranquilizers, and bed days—until the time of reemployment, and a small residual effect afterwards. The experience of having been unemployed was consistently associated with poor health outcome. However, when fault and no-fault were taken into account on the basis of individuals' own actions contributing to job loss versus circumstances beyond their control, those data showed that feeling at fault/ no-fault made no difference in the association between unemployment and physical illness, somatization, anxiety, and depression. Feeling at fault made the association between unemployment and poor health significantly greater for suicidal ideation, tranquilizer use, alcohol use, and bed days.

The authors calculated that people who experienced unemployment were between 54% and 68% more likely than the stably employed to report high levels of distress, levels severe enough to warrant professional intervention. The association of unemployment with alcohol use, suicidal ideation, and tranquilizers was dismissed as a selection effect, that is, a conservative approach in coding job loss as being outside the person's control. Poor health outcomes were possibly exacerbated by the realization that one was to blame for one's joblessness. The authors also found considerable variability in the extent to which reemployment could reverse the health-damaging effects of unemployment.

The effect of chronic stress associated with job loss and continuing unemployment was investigated by Fleming, Baum, Reddy, and Gatchel (1984), who looked at motivational consequences in subjects whose unemployment varied from a few days to four months; employed subjects were used as controls. Behavioral effects were measured by performance and persistence on an embedded figures task (EFT) and biochemical assessments were made from levels of catecholamines (epinephrine and norepinephrine) in the urine.

Unemployed subjects were found to differ from employed subjects on both physiological and behavioral indicators. They solved fewer puzzles and gave up sooner on the task. On comparing the subjects by dividing them into three groups depending on the length of time unemployed, those unemployed longer consistently had the higher level of urinary catecholamines.

Baum, Fleming, and Reddy (1986) used evidence of stress from catecholamine levels and behavioral difficulties from test performance deficits and hypothesized that one source of the stress was the noncontingency experienced between efforts at finding a job and the negative outcome of such attempts. Such negative outcomes were viewed as situations involving loss of control, increased reaction in efforts to reestablish control, followed eventually by learned helplessness as the length of exposure to the noncontingent settings increased.

Haney's (1979) review of the relationship of life events and coronary heart disease (CHD) identified unemployment as a major source of stress that impacted on the circulatory system and produced CHD. In his review, he noted such factors as stress (as perceived by the subject); the relationship of genetic factors, basic needs, and longings; earlier conditioning influences, life experiences, and cultural pressures, and mobility and migration. Haney summarized that behavior patterns, especially Type A behavior, environmental and social change, life events, and loss of employment should all be considered risk factors for CHD.

Haney found mixed results in the studies of the relationship between life events and cardiovascular disease, with retrospective designs indicating significantly high life-change units preceding the disease (Rahe & Lind, 1971; Rahe et al., 1976; Theorell & Rahe, 1971) and other studies showing no difference with prospective designs (Haynes et al., 1978; Hurst, Jenkins, & Rose, 1976).

Haney accepted the conclusion that social stress correlated with increased occurrence of various diseases and physiological changes. Although he listed a variety of explanations offered, he found criticism for each and preferred the unifying concept offered by Audy (1971). Audy felt that the difficulty in understanding health was the result of a tendency to regard health and disease as a continuum, as two ends of the same spectrum. Instead, he saw health as the ability to rally from insults—chemical, physical, psychological, and social. Insults may be of all kinds—positive, negative, excesses, deprivations, internal or external, etc.

Garfield (1980) related coronary disease to occupational stress by positing the idea of alienation as an integrating concept. Alienated labor resulted from the worker's lack of control over the work process, lack of investment in the product because of work conditions, and fragmented work relations. Thus, there were strong subjective feelings of powerlessness, dissatisfaction, and frustration, which contribute to coronary disease. Garfield suggested that chronic stress and alienation would be reduced as workers gained increased control over the process and product of their labor.

Kasl and Cobb (1982) criticized the cross-sectional approach in studies of unemployment because it tended to miss the complexity of the event and to provide misleading results that actually depended on when the measurements were taken. Their longitudinal study of two plant closings illustrated this concern in terms of both physical and psychological measurements. In physical measures, the authors reported that, on the basis of measures of days of complaint and days of disability, there were significant fluctuations over time but they could not be linked to employment–unemployment status changes. Analyses of cardiovascular risk factors such as blood pressure, serum cholesterol, cigarette smoking, and body weight showed no more risk for cardiovascular problems among men losing their jobs than among controls. The authors pointed out that most variables showed patterns of dynamic changes: between anticipation of plant closing and actual termination, the variables were reliably sensitive to differences between unemployment and prompt reemployment (especially changes in diastolic blood pressure and serum uric acid); between termination and four to eight months later, most subjects had returned to baseline levels. Apparently most men did not maintain a state of arousal or distress, but rather showed evidence of adaptation.

JOB LOSS AMONG PROFESSIONALS

For professionals, unemployment presents many of the problems and experiences found in job loss at all levels of work, but along with it, there are some unique experiences specific to the class of professionals, managers, technologists, and others at this level. Kaufman (1982) pointed out that unemployment among professionals is much greater now than it has been in previous decades and such condition can be expected to continue throughout the rest of this century. He related it to the rapid expansion of the supply of professionals in the United States along with a number of events that have diminished the demand, such as changes in national priorities, foreign competition, and the financial crisis in many of the cities.

Kaufman believes that work is probably more central to the identity of professionals than of other workers. When unemployment occurs, he estimates, as many as 40% experience psychological impairment extreme enough to require mental health assistance. Symptoms include low self-esteem, high anxiety, anomie, self-blame, depression, social isolation, anger, resentment, aggression towards others, psychosomatic disorders, occupational rigidity, professional obsolescence, low motivation to work, low achievement motivation, external locus of control, helplessness, and premature death from suicide or illness. These symptoms are expressions of devaluation of self-esteem, the diminishing of feelings of control, and emergence of feelings of helplessness.

Kaufman also believes that there is greater stress among those who have a graduate degree, particularly those involved in research and development work, stemming from the great material, intellectual, and psychological investment in developing their careers and in responding to the highly demanding nature of their work. The stages that the professional experiences at job loss are similar to those experienced by those at other work levels: shock, relief, and relaxation; concerted effort toward reemployment; vacillation, self-doubt, and anger as the frustration of not being able to find a job continues; resignation and withdrawal with diminished anxiety but a continuing sense of not being in control; and a loss of motivation.

Jacobson (1987) introduced some useful concepts in his discussion of meanings of unemployment among technical professionals. The stress that is felt may be interpreted from two models, transactional and transitional. Transactional stress occurs when demands tax or exceed the adaptive responses of the individual and the consequences of this imbalance negatively affect the individual's sense of well-being. Transitional stress stems from a relatively abrupt change in a person or her or his environment that affects the individual's assumptions about the world and her or his place in it. It is these assumptions that give meaning to the individual about events. When events challenge or change her or his assumptions, the individual's sense of meaning is undermined.

For Jacobson there was a direct relationship between financial resources and emotional states. Distinguishing between current income and capital consumption, he found that professionals described themselves in good shape when they had a surplus in terms of income over expenditures and had not dipped into savings or other reserves, thus maintaining a positive balance. Those who described themselves as managing were balancing between both, whereas those who were "in trouble" were exceeding and consuming their resources. Jacobson believes that researchers do not pay enough attention to the transitional stress experienced by professionals, such as unemployed engineers, scientists, and technical managers. Such people may experience "contextual threat" that contains the special meanings and implications of a job loss or vocational track that has been temporarily stopped or derailed.

SOCIAL SUPPORT AND UNEMPLOYMENT

In 1982 Mitchell, Billings, and Moos wrote a comprehensive review article on the relationship between social support and well-being, examining conclusions about direct effects of support on functioning, the indirect effects of support through its influence on environmental stressors, and the interactive effects of social support in buffering the individual from the maladaptive effects of stress. Although the article is general in terms of the relationship between support and well-being, the conclusions apply directly to the relationship of support to physical and mental well-being in the areas of work, job functioning, and unemployment.

The authors concluded that the evidence so far seemed to support the existence of all three effects—direct, indirect, and interactive support—on well-being, but because the area of support was complex, the results were not always consistent. There was ample evidence of a direct relationship between support and functioning, but the reciprocal influence of support and functioning on each other was still unclear. The authors suggested that social support might be used to promote well-being, such as enhancement programs for high stress groups like cancer victims, the frail, the elderly, the bereaved, and those undergoing stressful life transitions. More understanding is needed on how to build social networks that support identities and enhance self-esteem.

The authors also suggested that more specificity is needed in designing preventive interventions so that programs of support can be designed to offer specific types of support. Support may be time-limited, emotion-focused, or problem-focused, and outcomes may be either proximal or distal, or both. Social settings have been found to play a significant role in providing opportunities for the development of social ties. Characteristics of social settings can increase or decrease the likelihood that there will be groups that are at risk because of high stress and/or barriers against support.

A similar article by Wallston, Alagna, DeVellis, and DeVellis in 1983 reviewed the literature on social support and physical health, focusing on studies of illness onset, stress, utilization of health services, adherence to medical regimens, recovery, rehabilitation, and adaptation to illness. Like Mitchell, Billings, and Moos (1982), they concluded that the relationship of stress and social support to physical health still is not clear, perhaps because of the lack of more complex models and prospective research designs.

In general, the authors concluded that the research evidence supporting a direct link between social support and physical health is more modest than previous reviews had claimed. Apparently, there were different stages at which social support played more significant roles in mediating health outcomes than others. Social support was more than an environmental variable; personal characteristics as they affected access to, development of, and utilization of social support were important.

Wallston and colleagues felt that the term "social support" was too unwieldy to serve as a single meaningful construct.

Differentiation was needed among amount, nature, type, and source of support. In some instances, support implied beneficial involvement, whereas in others involvement was a burden. Social support during rehabilitation may even have created dependency rather than recovery.

The relationship between social support and physical health probably involved different processes at different stages of the health–illness cycle. At points throughout the cycle, from relative well-being through illness onset, health service utilization, adherence to regimen, adaptation to chronic illness, and so on, the process by which social support operated as well as the amount, type, or social support that was optimal may have differed. What was needed were actions that clarified contingencies, added predictability, reduced feelings of noncontrol or increased feelings of control that have been shown to mitigate the undesirable effects of unpredictable, uncontrollable events. Social support should contribute to such actions.

A significant article by LaRocco, House, and French (1980) explored the relationship between on-the-job stress and on-the-job strain among a wide range of occupational groups. The authors focused on the stress and strain found on the job rather than on the stress occurring with unemployment. They defined job stress as the conditions at work, role conflict, and other factors, whereas job strain was defined as the satisfaction from work and personal reactions to the job. Both factors—job stress and job strain—were considered to affect physical and mental health.

The authors used measures that obtained indices of stress, indices of strain, and measures of support from supervisors, co-workers, and families of over 2,000 workers from 23 occupational groups. Results indicated that support could buffer the relationship of perceived job stress and job strain on individual psychological well-being. The presence of support, however, did not buffer perceived job stress or job strain. Job-related sources of support had direct effects rather than buffering or indirect effects on job-related stress and strain. On the other hand, general health outcome was affected by a wider range of sources of support and the effects were more likely to be buffering effects than direct effects.

The authors suggested that the direct effects of support were beneficial for job-related stress or strain regardless of degree of stress experienced. As the degree of stress increased, more support was marshaled and was used as a buffer against increasing stress. If stress was low, support may not even have been used. The support that was mobilized would most likely have been used for mental health symptoms, or affects like depression and anxiety. Such symptoms are often viewed as psychosocially caused and therefore amenable to psychosocial support. On the other hand, job strain was seen as normal by most people, and support was not ordinarily marshaled for it. The more specific the stress and strain, or, for example, the more work-related, the more likely it is that specific or work-related support would have an impact. Familial sources of stress and strain, however, would probably be more affected by sources of support from family or intimate relatives and friends. This is very significant since job loss disrupts the availability of support systems.

Gore (1978) hypothesized that support would buffer the health effects of involuntary job loss. She was able to test her hypothesis on the employees of two different companies that were about to shut down their plants, one in a large city and the other in a small rural community. In addition, she used controls from similar plants in which her subjects remained employed.

Measuring the subjects at five stages—six weeks before, at termination, six months after, and one year and two years afterwards—she found that the physical measure of cholesterol level peaked for both unemployed and control subjects at stage two, termination. Both groups dropped by stage three, six months afterwards. However, the rate then stayed up for those who continued to be unemployed and unsupported by stage five, two years later. The rate had gone down for all those who were supported even though unemployed, but the rate stayed up for those unemployed and unsupported. Reported illness symptoms for unemployed and unsupported increased through stage two, and dropped with reemployment by stage three. Those who were unemployed but were effectively supported showed insignificant fluctuation throughout.

Depression was greatest among those who were unsupported, regardless of level of employment throughout the entire period of study. There were fewer abnormal changes for those who reported support during the early stressful changes, more self-blame was reported among the unsupported, and the unsupported consistently felt greater economic deprivation.

Gore's (1978) results were essentially the same as those of Kasl and Cobb (1982), in their study of the longer-term effects of plant closing on physical health. One plant was in a metropolitan area and the other in a rural area. They found that social support interacted with other variables in a complex way, specifically between phases one and two, preclosing and closing, with decreasing levels of serum cholesterol being much more associated with lower levels of social support in the urban setting and higher levels of support available in the rural setting. Diastolic blood pressure changed considerably in the early stages and relatively little in later stages. Serum uric acid was related to employment status between phases one and two, but not in later stages. Norepinephrine rates were not so much an indicator of impact as a predictor of the length of subsequent unemployment. In serum cholesterol, the biggest increase was found for men who experienced both unemployment and many job changes, and the biggest decrease was seen for those who experienced prompt reemployment and few job changes.

Atkinson, Liem, and Liem (1986) explored in depth the question of whether unemployment influenced quality and availability of social support resources. They also looked at the way in which support mediated changes and whether or not the stress-buffering hypothesis was valid. They studied families in Boston, half of whom were unemployed and the other half employed; half were blue-collar and the other half white-collar. The families were interviewed four times—two, four, seven, and 12 months following job loss. However, data were available only for the two- and four-month periods because most of the workers had become reemployed.

In general, unemployed workers, especially blue-collar workers, reported less support than employed respondents at both interviews. However, social supports of the reemployed were reported as increasing, whereas those of the unemployed were reported to be decreasing by the time of the second interview.

As hypothesized, the continuously employed had larger social networks than the reemployed, and the latter's networks tended to be equal in size or nonsignificantly larger than those of the continuously unemployed. There was a difference, however, among the networks of all three groups. The continuously unemployed, as well as the reemployed, added and dropped more members than did the employed controls. For the continuously unemployed, network additions were mostly new friends and relatives, and losses were of co-workers and old friends; for the reemployed, the changes were mostly additions of new friends and losses of old friends.

Duration of unemployment and marital quality were not significantly correlated when white-collar and blue-collar workers were grouped. However, white-collar workers with short periods of unemployment reported an increase in marital quality. Longer-term unemployment resulted in more negative reports. Similarly, information, advice, and concrete services were reported as decreased by white-collar workers who were unemployed for shorter periods of time. Frequency of contact with network members declined significantly over time for blue-collar workers only. This reflected more frequent contact with network members for the blue-collar workers who were unemployed for short periods, and declining frequency of contact with network members for blue-collar workers whose unemployment persisted.

Apparently, unemployment disrupted marital and family support, which was reported as less for unemployed workers than controls over both interviews. The longer the unemployment, the greater was the marital strain, especially in the white-collar group. It appeared that these men relied more heavily on people outside the immediate family for advice and information as well as for concrete services. They also received help from a greater number of helpers for each problem. The opposite was true of white-collar men whose unemployment was of short duration. These persons reported better marital quality and less reliance on outside support over time.

For all unemployed families, cohesion, marital support, and spouse role performance declined over time regardless of the duration of unemployment. Marital support indicators were most responsive to change, whereas social network measures showed little change. The strongest explanation for the above was the husband's reaction to the job loss, with his level of hostility, depression, and total symptoms accounting for most changes in social support. In addition, his anxiety, overall unhappiness, and negative mood influenced changes in family cohesion. The findings suggested that job losers tended to alienate the significant non-kin members of their social networks rather than their family members.

Atkinson, Liem, and Liem (1986) also indicated that it was important to note the time at which the level of support was measured because it varied. Some aspects appeared to deteriorate with continued unemployment, whereas others occurred at different periods. The authors pointed out that the stress-buffering process was different when there was a couple involved because there was an impact on the spouse who was severely distressed by her or his partner's reactions, and this distress then became a significant second source of stress for the unemployed person. It was, therefore, much more appropriate to assume that stress was mediated through networks of interdependence, such as family, work shift, or even community.

Revicki and May (1985) explored the relationships among stress, support, locus of control, and depression in a sample of over 210 physicians. Although not unemployed, the physicians were considered to be under continuous occupational stress as a result of their professional demands. The research focused on the possible mediating effects of locus of control and social support on stress and mental health among the physicians.

Age was found to be significantly related to peer support, locus of control, and depression, with older physicians possessing more supportive peer relationships than their younger colleagues. They also felt more personal control over their general environment, probably the result of longer-term experience. The lack of significant relationships among peer support, occupational stress, and depression may have been due to the nature of the physician's work. Most family physicians in private practice perform work activities independently, having little interaction with other physicians even in group practice.

The authors summarized their findings on support by stating that the study found occupational stress among physicians impacting directly on depression. This relationship was mediated directly by family support and indirectly by the influence of locus of control on stress and familial social support. Locus of control related directly to mental health. An indirect relationship was also found, suggesting that individuals with an internal locus of control may cognitively appraise stressful events and act directly toward these events in a way that enables them to cope more effectively with them. One way was to mobilize social support resources to help moderate the occupational stress.

COMMUNITY RESPONSES TO JOB LOSS

In general, health care providers have been very slow to respond to the human cost of unemployment (Liem, 1983). In earlier years there was little evidence that local health services, or the affected union, had adequate knowledge of the multiple hardships faced by job losers. Providers did not even have a procedure for obtaining information about employment status at the time of initial contact and were unaware of the extent to which unemployment was affecting service needs in the areas from which their patients came. In addition, those who lost their jobs were often hesitant to turn to outsiders for help. This was understandable in that getting by on one's own was at least one way to salvage some sense of self-esteem and dignity from the job-loss experience. On the other hand, at least some of the workers were aware that they needed counseling, although most families felt that they could not or would not ask for this kind of help.

The issue of self-blame was often involved in this situation. Therapists invariably approached the problems from a traditional therapeutic point of view and would worsen them by looking for ways in which the person was responsible for her or his job loss or poor health. In effect, unemployed workers who were already susceptible to self-blame found this orientation reinforced, despite the fact that a plant closing was completely out of the realm of their influence.

Responses from the community to job loss, plant closing, and unemployment have appeared in many different forms. Popay (1982) described a number of local responses to unemployment from self-help groups, trade unions, churches, professional organizations, mental health agencies, university placement centers, concerned citizens, and others. Sometimes actions were taken separately; often they were conducted by several resources working together. The programs vary depending upon the objectives, the population served, the subpopulations present, and concern over adverse effects of unemployment, including potential political ramifications.

Institute for Labor and Mental Health

The Institute for Labor and Mental Health, established in 1977 in Oakland, Calif., has been conducting job-related stress counseling among various groups of workers for a number of years, concentrating on combatting the self-blame tendency (Lerner, 1985). The Institute conducts occupational stress groups with a preventive focus on class and social dynamics, and externalization of the participant's anger. The Institute's rationale has been that an individual's anger over, for example, a plant closing and the resultant job loss is internalized and is responsible for much of the worker's health problems, both physical and emotional. Effort is directed toward helping people understand that their world is not a result simply of the choices they have made, but that the class options available to them and the class structure of the society as a whole have very much shaped their individual lives.

Work problems have been linked with community and family situations on the assumption that there is a relationship between family life and stress that people face at the workplace. The Institute is critical of traditional mental health services because they have tended to place responsibility for change on the individual and for leading workers to believe there was a wider range of individual choices available to them than was actually true. The Institute has related this assumption to a characteristic of society today—"surplus powerlessness." Powerlessness is both psychological and social. Within the labor market, surplus and real powerlessness mutually reinforce each other. The Institute conducted occupational stress groups to overcome the distrust and resistance people have to working together, and to combat surplus powerlessness. Shop stewards were selected and trained as agents of destigmatization in order to make it possible to discuss health issues at work. Massive advertising and media outreach were used to publicize programs, and the community was involved in day-long conferences.

An extension of the philosophy of the Institute for Labor and Mental Health is presented by Garfield (1980), who based his argument on the principle that people experienced increased stress when they lacked control over the situation and over the consequences of their own activities, a characteristic of industrial plant operation. The answer lay in the promotion of worker control. Productivity rises as workers assume more control over labor processes. Socialist programs can promote efficiency by changing wasteful and irrational socioeconomic conditions endemic to capitalism. A socialist transformation, essentially more worker participation and control in the industrial area, would reduce the sheer quality of labor time that society currently was requiring to sustain a given level of material culture at a given level of industrialization and technological capacity. Garfield (1980) stated: "With more people sharing a smaller aggregate work load, and with the transformed social relations and insensibilities that this entails, meaningful and satisfying work would more readily become an end in itself, rather than an occasional means of increasing productivity" (p. 559).

Community Mental Health Centers and Agency Interventions

Buss and Redburn (1983) found the problems encountered by mental health centers in a response to a plant closing in Youngstown, Ohio, were difficult because there were so few precedents. Although state and federal governments could be supportive in providing information on what other communities had done, the authors felt that each community must depend primarily on itself and develop its own resources. In Youngstown several services were provided, such as: a drop-in center to promote contact with workers and make referrals; a community mental health liaison that also provided outreach contacts; extension of the hours for the community mental health center (CMHC) to include evening hours; a community outreach organization that brought together experts and interested persons in the community; community education that was offered by various mental health programs; agency coordination and in-service training; and a crisis intervention service.

However, terminated workers made very little use of the available mental health services. Only 22 workers sought the services of the drop-in center set up in a local union hall, making the operation of a liaison function in the center all but useless. The crisis intervention center was the only program that received a large number of clients in need of services immediately after the plant closing. Not one manager or white-collar worker or her or his spouse sought services from one of the CMHCs. The blue-collar steel workers and their families did use the service of the CMHC: the wives were more likely to come in than the workers themselves; black and ethnic minorities came in relatively little. Massive emergency supplemental funding for mental health did little to affect the number of mental health services that were provided to the workers. An alcohol clinic in Youngstown yielded no information on the hypothesis that alcohol abuse was increasing in the community.

Many of the workers who did use the mental health center were unhappy with it. Only half reported satisfaction with the way they were treated and about 10% said that they were not treated with proper respect. In addition, many staff workers in mental health agencies were not familiar with services offered by other agencies. Workers were often misdirected and would become so frustrated that they simply dropped out. Many full-time workers had never been unemployed and were not comfortable dealing with public agencies, staff, and bureaucratic routine. Most workers wanted jobs from the service systems and were not interested in changing their lifestyles or accepting lower-status employment.

As alternatives to the formal system, approximately 20% of the workers indicated that they sought help from immediate family and other close relatives. Another 10% turned to the bank or finance company, and friends were contacted by an additional 11% to 12%. Greatest reliance was placed by workers on their immediate families and other close relatives. For a great many, unemployment seemed to bring out resourcefulness, whereas others did not seem to be able to cope either in the formal or informal helping system or on their own.

Various reasons were advanced for the low use of the mental health and human services. One explanation was the lack of need in terms of psychopathology. About 94% of the steel workers reported that they had never considered visiting a mental health agency, and 92% reported that they saw no need for that kind of service. Obviously, it is up to the mental health agencies to identify the needs and to develop ways of offering services in such a way that they will be used. Also, the mental health agency must work out some procedure for destigmatizing their agency and their services. Buss and Redburn (1983) concluded from their experience that though community mental health agencies may not become the primary source of services for unemployed workers, they might best serve as a catalyst for effective action.

Thompson (1983) reported the formation of a coalition in the Chicago area from suburban health systems agencies, the Cook County Department of Public Health, Park Forrest Health Department, and Health Partners of South Cook County. Their practical purpose was to gather data relevant to the newly unemployed and to suggest services and responses to whatever needs emerged. The effort focused on helping the health service by raising the level of awareness of the gaps in service; establishing a coordinated referral service with the county medical society and local hospital; publishing information for the unemployed on how to obtain free or low-cost care; developing workshops that teach the unemployed about maintaining health and locating central services; and pressuring state and federal government for legislation to provide insurance for those out of work.

Union-Based Programs

In England, unemployed workers' centers were established by the Trade Union Centers to provide services for the jobless (Popay, 1982). The objectives were to provide shorter-term needs, such as advice and counseling, information and support, education, representation, and recreation, as well as longer-term needs, such as job search and employment creation. Within two years there were 140 such centers in operation, funded primarily by the Trade Union Center, with a wide range of activities, including information, advice and counseling, education, arts representation, organization and facilities for children, cookery, and sports.

Drennen (1988) described a union program developed after a company closed its plant in Chicago. Stress management presentations were provided in union-sponsored, half-day workshops, with information on budgeting, dealing with creditors, unemployment benefits, retraining opportunities, and other help. Support groups, meeting weekly, discussed and sought out retraining opportunities through the union, discovered health insurance options, and educated one another on the status of their pension and on procedures for obtaining unemployment benefits. Discussions were held on such topics as a productive daily routine, knowing and communicating work skills and personality strengths, maintaining self-confidence, persistence in job seeking, and handling job interviews. In general, the group moved from having anxiety about being unemployed to making decisions about the future and stepping into various new life routines.

The union endorsement of the social services for the union workers and the outreach that began when the factory was closed were essential in helping the unemployed to develop the skills in coping with their job loss. Drennen recommended strongly that social service agencies in the community build relationships with labor leaders with whom workers have been familiar and on whom they have relied in the past as a way of increasing the utilization of social services and ensuring early intervention in the special crises of the unemployed.

One of the unique methods for relieving the stress of job loss was the formation of an "unemployment union" in response to needs of unemployed workers in Chicago (Schaps, 1983). When the mills along Lake Michigan closed, followed by deterioration of the community, the unemployment union was formed to focus directly on meeting the immediate needs of the workers. Organized like traditional unions with similar terminology and structure, it acted as a clearinghouse for part-time and shorter-term jobs, helped members negotiate contracts with potential employers, and tried to match service requests with the most appropriate union member.

A number of programs to increase skills and build solidarity within the group were developed. Not only was help offered in finding employment but efforts were made to foster spiritual and physical well-being along with community ties. Immediate needs of the unemployed worker were met by providing a directory of women's health services that would furnish adequate health care; also, an emergency food pantry was set up, security escort was made available for elderly residents, and

Al-Anon and Alcoholics Anonymous programs were offered.

Along with medical and physical health care, nonmedical services were instituted to improve health status. Teams sent to apartments to observe hazardous living conditions offered counseling on health problems, and the reduction of safety hazards. Environmental problems such as the presence of lead-based paint; porches, railings, and stairways in need of repair; need for pest control; and yards or lots requiring cleanup were identified. A nurse practitioner from the local county hospital provided immediate medical attention in an effort to avoid unnecessary hospital visits.

Corporate Programs

Popay (1982) sees a strong role for corporate management and industrial involvement in reducing the physical and mental health problems after job loss. One of these programs has been described by Beckett (1988). The program focused on mitigating the well-known negative effects of financial distress by paying attention to reducing economic loss and the loss of health and retirement benefits. When the company recognized that it would be necessary to close one of its plants in Washington, a two-year phaseout was initiated. The unions were informed and they bargained successfully for a closeout contract for their members that provided severance benefits, early retirement, and transfers to other plants. In addition, the corporation and plant management developed several programs, including stress management and career continuation seminars and employee and preretirement counseling. Plant personnel who were trained in the dynamics of separation and grief, along with recruited gerontologists, conducted sessions inside the plant. A firm that specialized in successful closings was hired to administer the plant shutdown.

Data were obtained before the plant was closed from employees aged 52 and older, and again a year later from similar respondents. Results indicated that the mental health of the older workers was not severely affected. Anxiety occurred only before the closing and not at the second data collection a year later, which indicated that the workers had experienced anticipatory anxiety rather than reactionary anxiety. Reemployed men seemed to have the highest anxiety level, suggesting that the anticipation of changing jobs was more stressful for them than either retirement or unemployment. The most plausible explanation for the lack of greater negative mental health effects on the workers seemed to be the company-sponsored programs and the reemployment of one-third of the sample. Income for many workers actually increased in the year following closing. Economic hardships were prevented by early retirement, alternate reemployment, and severance and layoff benefits.

Beckett (1988) concluded that it was important to advocate proactive economic support. Unions should include in their contracts provisions for phaseout programs, severance and mass layoff benefits, and extension of medical benefits after a closing. Closing a plant in phases rather than abruptly, giving advance notice, providing programs such as stress management, teaching national job search skills, and advancing early retirement to help workers appraise their options all helped. There was a relatively high utilization rate for accessible and relevant services, with programs held at the plant and on company time.

Stresses from repeated relocations have been identified in a profile called the "mobility syndrome" (Anderson & Stark, 1988). It includes depression, deterioration of health, little community involvement, strong dependency on the marital relationship for emotional satisfaction, a significant rate of alcoholism, pervasive feelings of social anonymity, diffusion of individual responsibility for social acts, destructive aggression, marital discord, and a high divorce rate. The families are stressed by the loss of support networks and valued persons and things, by the acquisition of greater role burdens, and by the interruption of personal growth and development. Teenagers seemed to be most adversely affected by geographical moves even under the best of conditions.

The strategies developed by the company for reducing the stress included transition counseling before and after the move, to help individual family members and the family as a unit to develop realistic expectations of the move. Counseling promoted the understanding of the impact on children, motivations for and against the move, and the process of phase adjustments.

The employee assistance programs (EAPs) have provided another strategy for the corporations. The EAPs, in cooperation with middle-level management, have developed methods to advocate corporate policies that significantly affect the lives and concerns of employees and their families. In the past ten years, there has been a rapid expansion of EAPs from fewer than 900 in the early 1970s to more than 5,000 in 1980. Family members, as well as employees, receive services. The EAPs offer ongoing counseling, biofeedback, stress management, and self-help or support groups for employees. EAPs may also develop the latest and most effective educational, promotional programs through interfacing with other company computer systems and developing computerized health-risk appraisals.

Other employers have met some of their social responsibilities in different ways. British Steel Corporation, for example, set up an enterprise trust concerned with training, retraining, and job creation. Pilkington Glass responded in a similar way by encouraging the development of small enterprises, and Standard Oil of Ohio offered career placement programs for spouses of workers who were relocated (Popay, 1982).

Mixed Resources

Of most interest are those programs that have drawn on a variety of resources for assistance in response to job loss. Sometimes there has been great ingenuity in forging excellent help out of a combination of resources.

In 1975 the MN industries announced a phaseout of operations in the Great River, Mich., plant. What followed was an innovative social experiment that combined management, union, university, and community representatives in a temporary interorganizational system. The coalition was formed because of the concern that the available social service agencies in the Great River area would not be able to coordinate activities effectively to deal with the unique constellation of problems caused by the sudden large-scale unemployment in the community. The coalition assumed responsibility for organizing the available elements into a coordinated attack on the problems expected to result.

The coalition was unique in that members of the University of Michigan faculty were enlisted to act as consultants and expert advisors and at the same time to conduct observations and develop theories about what was happening (Taber, Walsh, & Cooke, 1979). The program was initiated before the plant closed with the objective of facilitating the use of helping agencies after job loss and to evaluate the community and its response in the postclosure period. The problems that emerged were that the employees did not have information about possible helping agencies, did not recognize their own problems, did not seek assistance until it was too late, lost fringe benefits as well as wages, and had complexly interrelated problems. In addition, the employees lacked "bureaucratic competence," that is, the ability to deal successfully with bureaucratic agencies.

Comprehensive, coordinated services and proactive activities were needed in order for the community to provide for its members' service needs. Two major components were implemented: an organization to coordinate the community agencies and an in-plant counseling program to help workers define problems and contact appropriate helping agencies. The MN Community Services Council was formed as an interorganizational system with the express purpose of mobilizing community resources. In terms of theory, this Council was known as a "voluntary synthetic interorganizational community human services coordinating system."

The development of the Council went through three phases. In phase one, there was a period of initial rebuff and later acceptance of the community action team by several resources. Corporate support, for example, was not strong because their objectives for saving money conflicted with the efforts of the Council to reduce the human costs of the plant closing. In addition, elected representatives of the city of Great River were totally unsupportive. They were involved only in the longer-range business, economic, and political solutions, and the immediate problems seemed to have relatively little impact.

In phase two, the Council gathered information about the nature and severity of the problems faced by unemployed persons and identified specific community resources for those problems.

In phase three, the Council was refocused towards becoming a community resource by reconceptualizing it from a developmental, or resource-gathering, group to an operational resource group. Decision-making responsibility was consolidated in an executive committee consisting of the heads of all the committees and of current and future liaison groups, and the leadership duty shifted from the liaison group to a chairperson from the community.

Five main tasks were accomplished: (1) developing a domain consensus that did not take place until the Council began to shift its goals away from a "temporary industries" focus to a "continuing community" focus; (2) learning the extent of the problems and identifying available resources; (3) establishing linkages and at the same time protecting participants from threats to their boundaries; (4) developing an organizational structure at the same time that it carried on operations; (5) providing channels of communication to the developing organization, such as communication links between the in-plant counselors in the various agencies as well as among the agencies.

Taber, Walsh, and Cooke (1979) pointed out the irony in the fact that, although Great River already possessed comprehensive social services, the community could not have delivered the necessary response in a coordinated and proactive way before the plant shutdown. Had there been no crisis, organizers would have faced difficult problems in identifying relevant resources, gaining commitment from community leaders, and developing cooperation among the organizations.

Popay (1982) recognized that health services and professional groups have long been insensitive to and uninvolved in unemployment, but some change is now occurring. The Ohio Public Interest Campaign (OPIC)–Displaced Workers Project was made up of nonprofit organizations and citizens concerned with economic problems of the state. Individuals, trade unions, religious groups, and local politicians were enlisted by OPIC to help human service workers understand better and more effectively respond to special needs of displaced workers and their families. The Campaign facilitated development of worker support groups to help moderate the impact of the crisis. Professionals and unemployed workers were trained to respond to needs of unemployed persons.

OPIC became involved in plant closures through contacts with workers and union officials. It initiated plant meetings prior to a closure and helped the community to organize in forming groups to survey local job placement and training resources, to survey unemployed workers, to learn about situations and needs, to provide a directory of community agencies, to explore the feasibility of worker control of closing plants, and to support statewide plant closure legislation.

Programs for Professionals

Kaufman (1982) detailed some of the problems for professionals who have become unemployed and are faced with the prospect of seeking reemployment. Not belonging to a union means that for professionals the efforts are primarily individual. Kaufman classified job-search methods as formal and informal, with the former including private employment agencies, state employment services, and advertisements, and the latter involving use of personal contacts of any kind, including direct applications to employers. From a factor analysis of the methods used by unemployed professionals, Kaufman found five dimensions: (1) formal methods, such as private employment agencies, newspaper ads, professional journals, and the state employment service; (2) direct methods, such as application to employers in response to newspaper ads; (3) personal contacts, like friends and relatives and professional colleagues; (4) professional sources, such as professional societies, journals, and colleagues; and (5) no-fee services, such as former employers, outplacement services, college placement services, the state employment service, and national computer placement services.

Direct application was the most popular method, especially for older and more experienced professionals. It also was the most effective and efficient for professionals under less pressure to return to work. Newspaper ads ranked just under direct application in popularity, but they were not very effective or efficient. Personal contacts ranked almost as high as newspaper ads in utilization and were especially attractive for minorities. Private employment agencies ranked just below personal contacts, but were used primarily by higher-level and more educated professionals. College placement services ranked below private employment agencies and were classified as only moderate in terms of utilization. State employment service assistance was moderately used but it helped few professionals to find work. Professional journals and professional societies had moderate to low rates of utilization. Outplacement services by former employers were relatively unavailable and were concentrated in industries that experienced mass termination of professionals in cycles. National computer placement services were utilized by very few and with relatively little success.

Strategies that jobless professionals have used to improve their chances for reemployment have included geographic relocation, continuing education, retraining programs to transfer to a new career, and job counseling for professionals turned down after several job interviews with subsequent loss of confidence.

Underemployment occurred when the professional took a job at a lower level, primarily for security and as a temporary stopgap measure. For the most part, however, it was found to be damaging to long-range career growth, and ultimately to mental health.

Kaufman noted that it was possible for employers to initiate a number of strategies to avoid terminations. There were popular alternatives to termination, such as natural attrition or voluntary early retirement, but these were frequently limited. Employers could vary salary and working hours, with limitations on either or both, as effective alternatives to terminations. There were various ways in which work sharing could be used to reduce personnel costs without resulting in termination—for example, personnel could be reshuffled using internal transfers or retraining programs for new career positions. Employers also provided a variety of out-placement services directed primarily to minimizing the period of unemployment after termination. Services included providing information on job openings, job and career counseling, psychological assistance, preparing resumes, improving interviewing skills, and establishing various support services needed to carry out an effective job search campaign.

In the past, contributions by the mental health profession to the unemployed professional in dealing with problems created by job loss have been relatively limited. Most community mental health workers lacked adequate information on the impact of economic change, sometimes treating unemployment as a symptom. Kaufman recommended that mental health professionals should be trained with much more attention paid to economic factors. Self-help groups that incorporate assistance from mental health professionals have worked closely with the employment services and with community-oriented programs. Interventions by mental health services prior to job loss would be more effective. In order to minimize unemployment stress, notification of termination as soon as possible after the actual decision is made is important. Out-placement activities should be initiated simultaneously with notification of termination, along with provision of emotional and instrumental support for the activities.

Kaufman also recommended that mental health considerations should be incorporated into personnel practices, such as paying attention to potential reentry problems, providing for appropriate placement, assigning positions involving relocation with care, and providing retraining programs and career changes for those who have gone through a long job search but have not yet reached the final stage of withdrawal and resignation.

3

Displaced Worker Programs: A Community-Crisis Approach

PSYCHOSOCIAL INTERVENTION

This chapter describes a conceptual model of psychosocial intervention for displaced workers. The programs to which we shall be referring are the psychosocial interventions that include outreach, assessment, and individual and group counseling and that were offered to displaced workers participating in federally funded retraining and reemployment efforts.

Mental health services are often introduced into a community when an event such as a plant closing, disaster, or other larger-scale crisis arises. Some of these community-based crisis model programs have been only moderately successful because of low utilization of services. One reason for this is that responses to these stressors are transitory phenomena. The community is resistant to offers of help by mental health professionals because this implies the presence of mental illness. The initial approach to the affected community may be a preventive mode, such as outreach to victims. However, what takes place after this stage is still traditional, introspective, client-focused therapy and rarely situational and socio-psychologically focused interventions. One usually finds the latter in the treatment of stress-related illnesses, such as heart attacks, and self-destructive behaviors, such as suicide and substance abuse.

The goal of these psychosocial intervention programs is to serve as a supportive component to the retraining and reemployment process. The staff members participate in these processes of enforced change and attempt to ameliorate the psychological impact of sudden job loss on displaced workers. The community-based crisis model itself allows the professional to serve as an informal consultant during a time of organizational stress. It is a model readily adapted to community mental health centers and others not necessarily affiliated with an institutional setting. An affiliation with a social agency or other organization provides legitimacy, since publicly funded displaced worker programs generally emerge from the community mental health system, as is often the case in the industrial Midwest. Active participation in planning these efforts can thus enable the community-oriented mental health professional to influence the decision-making process. Such efforts often bring together professionals from a number of cross-cutting systems. There are, however, factors that inhibit the development of rapport, understanding, and shared trust. There is a perception, widely held by the public, that efforts developed by mental health professionals on behalf of displaced workers are stigmatizing. Administrators in the field of retraining and employment development often believe that such efforts should be limited to the disturbed clients. The displaced workers, who are themselves experiencing transitional stress, resist the mental health professionals' labeling of them as having emotional problems.

These factors contribute to the role conflict that emerges when the mental health professional participates in the planning and early implementation of these interventions. Although the displaced worker program may tap the resources of the mental health center, it may take place on-site in the affected community at the union hall, the plant, the community college, or other training location. These are sites that afford minimal identification of services as a mental health program. On the other hand, destigmatizing of the mental health image also brings with it the problem of legitimacy. Decentralization of these interventions may raise questions regarding the program's and professional's credibility to the client, the community, and the network of mental health and social service providers. The resolution of these legitimacy questions must lie within the credibility of the clinician's interactions with these constituencies, rather than in the profession itself. This renders the situation even more complex because clinical staff members will often become uncertain of their functions, which leads to perceived role ambiguity.

These role conflicts often have to do with perceiving the displaced worker as a patient, rather than a person in a transitional phase. Traditionally, mental health professionals treat troubled people, with their initial efforts being the performance of a diagnostic function and, more recently, the arrival at a diagnostic category. The inclusion in DSM-III (*The Diagnostic and Statistical Manual of Mental Disorders: Third Edition*) of post-traumatic stress disorders has helped to validate the impact of such transitional events as disasters, wars, and civil disorders on emotional functioning. The mental health system has been in crisis over limitations of service imposed by third-party providers and others, including Employee Assistance Programs. Prevention programs usually are given outside of this system of clinically based services and, therefore, are seen to be of secondary value by the more traditional therapist. It is important, therefore, to conceptualize work with the unemployed person as being within the domain of prevention. There is a concurrent need in these and other prevention efforts, as in the field of psychotherapy research, to document the effectiveness of the psychosocial interventions.

The possibility of establishing these programs has increased since personnel managers and middle management within the private sector in general have been exposed to and have become aware of mental health needs at the workplace. Employee Assistance Programs (EAPs) emerged initially from the alcoholism field and were designed to address employer concerns that result in such workplace-related behaviors as absenteeism, industrial accidents, and poor performance. Refer rals to these programs were part of a disciplinary action initiated by supervisory personnel. Self-referral to EAP services is an option now available to employees. Mental health services were a later addition to the EAP model and are still not included in all such programs. In major metropolitan communities, mental health crisis services have become a part of the employee benefit package in law enforcement and public safety agencies. The California Highway Patrol, for example, provides crisis services for all employees and 100% mental health coverage after five years of service. Workplace mental health education programs bring a preventive focus to such areas as parenting and family life, stress reduction, health promotion, and preretirement planning. What has been described are employee benefits negotiated by the union or used by employers as incentives or "perks" for recruitment and work force maintenance and stability.

Companies that support these efforts are likely to mobilize resources for their employees when layoffs and closures occur, although economic considerations may limit the extent of their participation in such efforts. Companies with EAP services are more apt to consider a preplant closure intervention as an option for their workers. Company management recognizes the need for an outside organization to provide such services as stress counseling and group-level interventions. Companies facing closure are confronted with the dissolution of the existing personnel and managerial structure. Since the EAP is viewed by management as the mechanism for resolving conflict for troubled employees, these services are not used as the vehicle for support and assistance for the work force at large during the transition to job loss.

The clinician who is accustomed to a case-finding approach will be familiar with the referral mechanism of the EAP, with the third-party payment structure of private insurance plans, and with the community mental health system. However, the relationship to the "client" in preplant closure intervention programs is at best precarious. The sanction to identify the troubled participant—that is, to conduct active case-finding within this setting—is not implicit in these programs. Mental health professionals in hospital settings find it difficult to apply their clinical skill. The case-finding that may occur at this stage, during the group-level interventions, is the recognition of disturbed individuals in need of mental health services, who have been functioning in their jobs. The immediate concern is the future employability of the troubled person who has thus far managed to adapt and who has been accepted within the workplace from which she or he is departing. When the participant seeks help, there is no dilemma. However, when the clinician recognizes extreme pathology, without the sanction to intervene, a strong internal conflict may emerge. Frequently, the only option available is to reiterate information within the group setting regarding trouble signs related to post-traumatic stress symptoms and available community resources. The clinician can share his or her concern regarding specific individuals with company personnel managers, though without disclosing confidential information. Although none of this information will surprise the enlightened personnel manager, the clinician's concern may reinforce the need for management to intervene on behalf of the troubled client. These actions by the company may occur as a result of altruism, but they may also take place in an effort to avoid worker's compensation and other disability claims.

The mental health professional must, therefore, approach his or her tasks with confidence, a clear sense of what can be done, and the value of the work. There is the concurrent need to view one's professional status as conferring worth on the services and the recommendations provided, because the mental health practitioner is frequently entering a world within which there is only partial acceptance of the validity of the intervention strategy. These attitudes, moreover, often interfere with collegial arrangements to the detriment of the client population. Because of these obstacles, the mental health professional must be clear on both the goals and the validity of the professional efforts. Working with reluctant systems may evoke feelings of anger and diminish one's motivation to continue efforts on behalf of the clients. These feelings of ambivalence in relation to the work are self-defeating. Just as we attempt to develop a sense of empowerment in the client, the mental health professional must never lose sight of her or his power and the ethics of the profession. This entails maintaining a balance in one's relationships with representatives of the various cross-cutting administrative systems.

The maintenance of balanced "peer" relationships with other professionals is necessary to prevent the development of a form of interaction commonly referred to as "one-down" or unequal exchange. Such ties are essential as well, so that the clients perceive the unanimity among the professionals assisting them. This role modeling helps clients understand the way in which diverse individuals and systems operate. The client caught in the nexus of bureaucratic oversights, for example, may play one system against the other as a way of discharging anger and frustration. Through strong internal ties among professionals in a team or service network, the clients will perceive the legitimacy of their points of view in a clear, direct manner. In this way, the clients' sense of self-worth is encouraged and the process necessary for self-empowerment to develop is initiated.

IDEOLOGICAL CONCEPTIONS OF THE HELPING PROCESS

A central concern in the delivery of community-based psychosocial interventions for displaced workers is the array of stigmatizing assumptions, images, services, and labels that are projected upon a working-class population. The worker population already recognizes that there are individuals with substance abuse and family problems within their ranks and they are sensitive to deviance as well. There is currently more familiarity with psychological therapy because of increased media exposure, through radio talk shows. Despite a commonsense awareness that the trouble caused by economic worries can affect their personal lives and emotional functioning, these workers will critically question the assumptions and efficacy of the clinical intervention. The mental health professional, traditionally trained, arrives with a carrying case of skills derived from the university and professional school, and holding the belief that psychotherapy is "the real thing." The term "stress counseling," on the other hand, carries less stigma because it is often seen within a social framework. The program model must reflect this sense that the external environment is the primary cause of the problem.

The community crisis model program often emerges from efforts by those in the mental health field to appeal to the special needs of an affected population. There is a semantic issue involved in using mental health labels to define the community-based program. Potential participants will not respond to a mental health term, such as "crisis counseling," and will even resist the less stigmatizing term, "stress counseling," and this often holds true in the case of larger-scale community events, such as disaster, sudden job loss, or other traumatic stressors. The suggested titles for displaced worker interventions—for example, "layoff assistance program" and "workplace liaison program"—emerged from earlier poor attendance at what was previously offered as "stress counseling" workshops. There was a noticeable change in attendance when these groups were renamed "career dynamics workshops."

Potential clients may hold attitudes towards mental health programs during the crisis of sudden job loss. This attitudinal set results in both the avoidance of any help and the belief that there is nothing psychologically or emotionally wrong. The very act of stepping forth and accepting help would, in their estimation, identify them as having pathology. Even though some of these individuals have previously utilized mental health services, these programs are not routinely sought by workers during layoff. They are often not seeking help for personal problems during the initial post-layoff period. They are, rather, requesting assistance for their immediate, material needs, and perhaps family and child problems. Because this population has a different frame of reference toward the program, the professional begins to develop a sense of mission or purpose that often lies outside the traditional mental health paradigm.

CASE

In the initial planning phase of an intervention at a food manufacturing company, negotiations took place with personnel department representatives and with mental health professionals regarding proposed services for the about-to-be-laid-off workers. They were enthusiastic and supportive of stress counseling as the key to a successful plant closure program. The personnel director was empathic to the workers' plight because he had interacted with them over time. He recognized that the workers were upset and uncertain and felt that it was the company's responsibility to help them. Management personnel were also sensitive and responsive to the psychological needs of the workers.

During the pre-layoff orientations, information was presented to the workers about the range of services available to them. At this point, it became less clear how stress counseling services would be made available to them because of the immediacy of their job loss and the company's policy regarding severance pay and other termination benefits. Coincidentally, the "sympathetic" personnel manager was transferred to another plant. The new personnel manager was more distant from the workers and more rigid regarding released time for workshop attendance. This created barriers to workers having access to supportive services during the pre-layoff phase. There was no active union participation, and advocacy on behalf of the workers by union officials was not provided. This became a major obstacle to implementing a stress counseling program because of a lack of mediating influences of representatives from a labor or governmental organization.

The counseling program consultant became a catalyst for organizational change by demonstrating an understanding of the company's administrative needs during the transition and the difficulties confronted by personnel department staff. The consultant became in this sense an ally to the process of change, albeit from a tangential position with relation to the organizational system. This was accomplished through brief, face-to-face meetings with the personnel assistant to develop trust and to establish common concerns. Discussions focused on strategies that needed to be developed collaboratively with management representatives and with allies from the work force, in order to smooth the way during this transition and to deliver effective services.

The first two group sessions at the plant for the workers to be laid off were poorly attended, the reasons being the previously mentioned management changes and the ambivalence of the new management team. The workers were not notified about meeting times, and there were schedule conflicts between stress counseling services and other job-search activities. The stress counseling team restructured the terms of service delivery for operational effectiveness. This meant producing and distributing printed materials, delivering announcements over the public address system, and creating an alliance with employee representatives. The alliance developed, in this case, with the personnel department assistant and the handful of individuals who attended the early workshops and who became advocates of the program.

This case illustrates the impact of the stress counseling team as a "presence," whose members observe the core issues within an organization, assess levels of tension, predict conflict areas, and provide support to others who are involved in the helping effort. On the individual level, the team members can help to recognize the trouble situations and perhaps forestall extreme behaviors within the affected population. In order, therefore, to deliver services, the team must operate on multiple levels within the system.

GROUP INTERVENTIONS

Group counseling is the primary intervention utilized in this program. The groups are task-oriented with a focus on specific content areas. The initial session begins with introductions. The leader(s) request that each participant in turn introduce him- or herself and share specific information with the group. This includes job history, length of employment, description of the job, and current job plans. The leaders interact in this process and also interject appropriate affective observations and comments on observed feelings of loss, anger, bewilderment, and self-blame. The leaders then clarify the agenda of the group sessions, explain the program goals and objectives of these group sessions, and present their perspectives and observations. These include reviewing issues relating to unemployment and stress, personal empowerment, the impact of loss, and coping strategies during this phase. The leaders also clarify the didactic focus of these groups, at the same time demonstrating, by modeling sensitivity and compassion, awareness of the personal struggles experienced by participants. This is a deliberate attempt to provide structure and to clarify participants' expectations. Presentation style is both informal and authoritative.

Group-level interventions are particularly effective in this process of objectifying the circumstances involved in losing one's job. These circumstances are externalized in a group setting when the victims of a layoff talk about the conditions in the company that led to the layoff. This opportunity to ventilate, reflect, and share perceptions and reactions to a common event is cathartic. To hear others express their feelings and interpret the objective reality of the event helps to reduce an individual's distortion and personalization of the event. This threefold process of (1) individual narration of the event, (2) description of reactions to it, and (3) coping strategies and individuals' plans for the immediate future provides the framework for self-empowerment. Learning from one's peers vicariously in a group setting corrects any distortion about the cause of the event. This process of peer learning both diminishes tendencies towards self-blame for having lost this job and facilitates exploration of options for dealing with loss and change.

Mini-therapeutic transactions incorporate the elements of the crisis intervention model: the hazard, the crisis, the adaptive coping strengths, and the individual's capacity to resolve the situation. Modeling this approach within the interchange encourages the participant to perceive the facilitator as a therapeutic agent. The use of nontechnical language to structure these transactions is essential.

The provision of information about community resources and the distribution of written materials are helpful in this group setting. When this information is disseminated in the group, with recommendations about effective help-seeking strategies, the displaced worker is more willing to accept the information and is less defensive about the implications of seeking help from community agencies. Since these individuals have not been traditional recipients of public entitlement programs and other community services, they have a very strong bias against welfare programs and those who receive social services. Blue-collar workers, in particular, stigmatize those groups as being less worthy and are offended by any inferences that they would, in the future, fall into these categories. When presenting such materials and information, the facilitator should suggest, "You may be able to help others by having this information handy." This type of remark also serves to empower the displaced worker as a helping agent to others in difficult situations.

OVERVIEW OF GROUP SESSIONS

The career dynamics groups modeled after Schein (1978) involve participants from a variety of work settings. The focus of the groups is: (1) human relations skills-building, including self-presentation, motivation, and self-esteem; and (2) coping skills during periods of transition, including training, job search, and reentering the workplace. The group sessions are held on-site at the workplace in the case of preplant-closing interventions or at assigned community locations, and become mutual support groups on how to cope successfully with stressful life transitions and their effects on health, motivation, and attitude. These groups are made up of workers from the same workplace and, in some instances, are heterogeneous groupings of displaced workers from a variety of companies.

The groups provide the framework for participants to discuss perceived obstacles in their training and job-search efforts, to recognize stress reactions, and to cope more effectively by enabling them to confront problem issues early on in the transitional period, including such substantive concerns as: (1) transition to a new job and workplace; (2) interpersonal relations on the job; and (3) development of initial contact with job placement staff regarding on-the-job and classroom training situations.

Session 1. The group begins with a round-robin introduction where participants state their names, occupation, length of employment, and future goals. The session covers the basic issues involved in transitional change and the importance of the following questions:

1. What are your goals? What obstacles would keep you from meeting your goals?
2. What new systems (e.g., state employment service, retraining institutions, placement agencies) have you entered recently? Have you dealt with them effectively or felt powerless in your relations with them?

The group facilitator then helps participants to focus on problem solving and on identifying personal strengths through discussion of the following topics: (a) overcoming personal barriers; (b) building self-esteem; (c) assessing self-worth; and (d) building confidence. The group enables individuals to develop insight regarding their situation through increased knowledge, peer support, and directed learning. The expected outcome is some change in perception of the participants' sense of mastery and self-efficacy in dealing with new situations and self-empowerment in working with systems.

Session 2. The group is asked to complete a stress/coping self-administered test developed by the State of California Department of Mental Health, entitled "Friends Can Be Good

Medicine." This process involves gaining insight through addressing the following questions:

1. What life events have you experienced within the past year? What are the present causes of stress in your life?
2. How do you usually cope with stress on the job? What coping strategies work best for you at home?
3. Who are the sources of support in your life? How effective are they in helping you through this present crisis?

The group then allows participants to discuss their own stressful situations, personal coping strategies (adaptive and maladaptive), and social network relations (identifying sources and examining their effectiveness). There is a brief discussion of the relationship between stress and physical and emotional illness, as well as the role of positive coping in preventing such illnesses. The group enables individuals to assess their human relations skills through increasing their knowledge of the networks of support that surround them, and emphasizing the importance of maintaining interpersonal ties during periods of transition through good communication, assertiveness, and effective listening. The expected outcome is some change in perception of the participants' social world, coping mechanisms, and human relations skills.

Session 3. The group is asked to develop a personal time line of goals, strategies, and expected completion dates for each goal. The process involves the development of realistic life-planning and decision-making skills by addressing the following questions:

1. What are your current needs and priorities? How do you plan to meet these needs, i.e., What is your "game plan"?
2. What is your step-by-step approach to planning and decision-making?

3. How will you follow through on your plans and decisions, i.e., How will you "get on course"?

The group facilitates a discussion of each participant's life
plans with respect to personal decision-making and time
management over the transitional period. The group enables
individuals to share information regarding job-search strategies,
ventilate their frustrations and hopes regarding their future,
and discuss, as well as role play, the situations that they
perceive as stressful yet necessary to an optimal outcome. The
expected outcome of this process is some change in perception of the participants' rational goals and priorities, anticipated
results, and the steps and procedures necessary for success.

With a team of two leaders, the possibilities for observation
and interaction are strengthened. The group seems to get out
of control at one time or another, with laughter and jesting,
teasing, and sometimes resistant silence. This model of group
intervention results in less resistance than previously observed
unstructured group interventions. They are less likely to be
perceived as being intrusive, as leaders do not make interpretations in psychological language or delve into their less-
conscious motivations. Participants attend these groups for
assistance in coping with stresses related to job loss and for
help in acquiring new employment. They have not made a
psychotherapeutic contract. The clinically trained leaders may
have difficulty with these more prevention-oriented groups,
unless they are clear about the process and goals. A leader's
clinical skills, such as insight into the thematic content of each
client, however, are necessary for the group process. These
groups are designed for functioning individuals, but there are
times when the groups include more deviant individuals. The
leader must use clinical judgment and skills to control disruptive and inappropriate behaviors within the group, by minimizing these behaviors and allowing unruly persons to ventilate
their feelings. There are times when these participants will require individual intervention, and occasionally requests for individual sessions are made; thus, it is necessary to maintain
liaison with community agencies.

The goal of the groups is to validate the individual's perceptions and experiences. The group leaders encourage the individual to ventilate his or her feelings and then to move to the next phase. Since the groups are structurally time-limited, the leaders need to reinforce the view that the individuals have strength from within themselves, from their peers, and from what is commonly called their support system. The displaced workers are encouraged to regard the group leaders as only the facilitators of self-exploration and decision making. Some participants seem to need more help from the leaders and others seek out social interaction. The leaders have the responsibility to encourage group members to utilize the services available to them from other helpers in the system, such as vocational counselors or personnel staff. The purpose of this strategy is to dilute the attachment to a group leader and to encourage the perception of a network of helpers in this reemployment effort. Similar to crisis group therapy, and other time-limited groups, the transference is minimized. The short-term nature of the alliance precludes fostering dependency upon the therapist/group leaders. Rather, the goal of these interventions is for the individuals to tap their strengths and mobilize previously developed coping mechanisms to deal with this crisis.

Many working people, particularly men, have difficulty understanding that the emotional reactions they are experiencing are shared by others. Working women appear to find it easier to provide emotional support to each other. The working-class male's inhibited ability to talk with his peers about his feelings of loss increases his sense of emotional isolation.

CASE

A Black, male laborer in his mid-30s, who worked in the food processing industry, escorted his wife to the group with the expectation that he would not stay for the session. He hovered near the doorway while members of the group encouraged him to join in. The group leader lightly said, "You are welcome to join us, and you don't have to say anything if you don't want to." He reluctantly sat at the edge of the group, and when it was his turn, introduced himself shyly. As the session progressed, he talked about his own work experience. He presented himself to the group with self-confidence in his wage-earning ability. Statements such as, "I've always been able to get a job, and I'll always be able to," reflect his certainty about his competence. When queried about the kind of work he would like to do, he became reflective and talked about work that he enjoyed in the past, specifically landscaping. The group leader validated his competence by saying, "You've really done a lot of things" and concretely informed him about a training program for tree trimmers. The group focus then shifted from him to others, and later on in the session, he spontaneously participated and sought out information from the group leader. His wife, who had also stayed, spoke about her own employment training goals, namely, to become a medical assistant, and also shared in the economic fears of some of the other group members. One of the other women reassured her that with such a self-confident husband, she would be able to achieve her career goals. Her husband then became supportive of another man in the group who was expressing his ambivalence towards retraining options. Thus, the process of mutual disclosure and peer support enabled him to begin to get a sense of his independent strengths and sense of self-empowerment.

The case illustrates the type of orientation toward the event and the individual approaching a crisis that the members of the team must have in order to serve the target population effectively. The example demonstrates the issue of intrusiveness as it is perceived by blue-collar workers who tend not to be psychologically introspective. Interactions with this population need to be conducted in a manner that respects their reality situation. Blue-collar workers differ from those characterized as the "worried well," in that they do not perceive themselves as troubled people, despite the fact that many of them are already struggling with family and other problems. The external event of job loss requires that individuals be able to tap strengths that will help them through the transition; for some of these individuals, problems do arise because of inadequate coping skills. Since they do not identify these problems as psychological ones, and in reality they may not be, the intervention techniques must be sensitive to this reality. This includes knowledge of the conceptual boundaries of the population, that is, the rules of appropriate forms of conversation. For example, during an initial interview the question, "Are you having any problems?" would be interpreted as relating to material or financial problems.

DISCLOSURE AND TRUST-BUILDING

There is a major difference between working with individuals during a mass layoff and working with these individuals within a group setting. What occurs in individual psychotherapy is gradual trust building that facilitates growth. This also occurs in traditional group psychotherapy. However, in these transitional groups for displaced workers, the opportunity and time for trust building is frequently not available. Trust has to derive from the credibility that the leaders convey from having worked with others in this same situation and their familiarity and understanding of the workplace, the jobs, and the nature of the stressful event. These components help reduce the barrier between the group leaders and the individuals in the group. These groups are conducted in commonsense language, on the workers' turf, and with a minimum of social barriers between professional and client. This is a conscious attempt to build a trust relationship quickly. It is important for the group leaders to recognize limits in the interactions and to keep a constant watch that the boundaries between the individuals are never violated.

Upon entry into the group, the leaders must establish a neutral stance toward both the company and, when appropriate, the labor organization. To be most effective, the facilitators must be viewed as potential advocates and a source of information. The leaders must be directive in regard to eliciting from the displaced workers concrete information about who they are, what they do, how long they have been employed, and what their current activities have been with regard to job search and planning for the future, that is, choosing a training program or entering early retirement. For displaced workers to speak before a group of their peers about these matters is frequently accompanied by embarrassment, bravado, and other postures. This is an unfamiliar role for these workers. Thus, it is helpful in the group process to start out with the less emotionally laden subjects, which will allow individuals to experience the group as nonthreatening and thereby facilitate trust building. The leaders use this opportunity to interject comments and to build on the camaraderie within the group and to become a part of a familiarizing process.

Traditional group dynamics principles can be applied to the transitional stress group only to a limited degree. Although facilitation may be restricted to setting goals for each session, very highly developed leadership skills are necessary. Unlike a therapy group, direction and control need to be exerted. It should be kept in mind that the most outspoken member of the group is often the least representative. This individual may openly express opinions regarding the layoff, such as the unequivocal support of the company and its largesse, but often is perceived as a "blowhard" or a clown, or in other ways as being unrepresentative of the point of view of the majority of the participants. This person is rarely a leader or spokesperson.

The issue of intrusion upon the individual client's sense of privacy must be constantly kept in mind. In naturally occurring groupings in a workplace, close peers often talk informally about personal issues, including relationships and other intimate details and problems. Talking about private issues in a public forum, such as in a transitional support group, however, can serve as the client's rationale for resistance and dropping out. It is for this reason that the immediate reality of job loss and coping with the stressful transition from the content of group discussions. The recent success of psychological talk shows on the radio, by contrast, may lie in the anonymity of the caller, so that a person's sense of shame is diminished as his or her identity is concealed. Popular psychology books may also have familiarized the public with talking about intimate problems and with the kinds of psychological explanations provided by media-oriented helping professionals. Self-help groups, such as Alcoholics Anonymous, have also provided a language for dealing with introspection and emotional control.

INDIVIDUAL NARRATIVE AND GROUP PROCESS

In the initial phase of the group process, participants relate their individual stories by recounting the circumstances that resulted in their unemployment. Various reactions can be observed within the group, ranging from apparent disinterest to expressions of support. This first exercise can be very stressful, as it forces the individual to present the current life situation before the group. Even though all participants share a common concern, their individual reactions to the stressor vary. The group leaders encourage a dynamic interaction within the group in this first session, so that the group itself becomes the helping agent.

The leaders and the group learn about the particular circumstances of each participant's work life and the events surrounding job loss. The individual has the opportunity to tell her or his story and to be heard in a respectful, interested way by the group leaders. Other group members, who may be from the same workplace, may at times disagree with the way the "tale is told." The group leaders are receiving new information regarding the situation of the participants and their workplace, and may ask for clarification regarding the circumstances. The participant is the "expert" regarding these circumstances, and the atmosphere created is much less threatening since each person is seen as presenting a valid depiction. When a layoff is impending, co-workers have many opportunities to commiserate and to evaluate their feelings about their situation. After layoff, these opportunities diminish; family members and friends are rarely receptive to repetitive recounting of the circumstances. The group presents an opportunity for retelling to patient listeners.

The group serves, therefore, as the key medium of supportive intervention during the transitional phase of job loss for a number of important reasons. The displaced worker experiences the threatened loss of the familiar occupational environment and that of the personal ties to co-workers. The worker benefits, however, from the collective support that a group of peers can offer during this period of transition. Group members have shared concerns, and the support group enables peers to verbalize their common anxieties and thereby validate them. Common themes may emerge when individuals share these accounts of the effect of sudden job loss on their lives, sources of livelihood, and sense of well-being. Such collective attempts at sense-making help those in crisis to reestablish their personal boundaries and to reformulate a coherent perception of their world.

4

The Mental Health Consultation Model and Displaced Worker Programs

DYNAMICS OF THE MENTAL HEALTH CONSULTATION PROCESS

There are many different models for mental health interventions for displaced workers, the reason being that control of the psychosocial intervention program lies outside the full control of the mental health system. The key players are within the employment development and job placement organizations in both the public and private sectors. The reason is self-evident—both industry and the labor union are primarily concerned with returning their constituencies to paid employment. The emphasis, therefore, is upon preemployment preparation, such as job-search workshops, classroom and on-the-job training, and job clubs. The mental health professional may assume the role of a consultant to, and perhaps a mediator in, the process of interagency and intraprogram facilitation.

According to Caplan (1964, 1970), the mental health consultation model focuses on program development or administrative problems. It is a "consultee-centered case consultation" model, namely, one that focuses on cases or clients of the consultee. The objectives of the model are: (1) to improve the work effectiveness of the consultee, which subsequently helps clients' performance and psychological development; and (2) to enhance the understanding of the psychological issues involved in the case and, thereby, alleviate the emotional blocks that may be interfering with such an objective understanding.

The preparatory stage of the consulting process involves obtaining information on the formal organization and informal power distribution of the consultee system—the company, government agency, or training center—through materials published by that organization, newspaper accounts, informal contacts, and interviews with personnel. The consultant thereby develops an understanding of the structure of the consultee organization that may help to delineate system barriers to the process of change. The key issue during this stage is the examination of the history of one's own relationship with the consultee organization, that is, previous experiences and preconceptions that may affect attitudinal issues as they emerge during the consultation.

The entry stage of the consulting process involves formally initiating contact with the consultee, accepting the existing relationships, and gaining the respect of the peers within the organization. The consultant must develop a sense of intimate familiarity through direct and participant observation of organized activities. The consultant begins to clarify her or his role and, at the same time, engages in reality testing of that system's defenses. The key issue during this stage is the avoidance of cooptation by the consultee as an ally during the internecine conflicts that characterize a system in crisis. The formal consultation stage in these displaced worker programs formed under legislated federal Job Training Partnership Act funding and administered by localized reemployment and retraining programs is indeed paradoxical. The mental health professional is a "consultant without portfolio" who is part of the process of change, yet lies outside of the system because of her or his professional identification. The mode of consultation is equally paradoxical, as the consultant must initiate an "informal interaction process" (Ketterer, 1981) in order to bring about formal changes in the consultee's organization. This process involves: (1) planning for program effectiveness; (2) identifying the potential problems in the consultee; (3) developing common modes of understanding these problems; (4) focusing on the stressors on the consultee; (5) clarifying concepts of strain with the consultee; (6) recommending options and strategies; and (7) assisting the consultee in overcoming resistances and attitudinal blocks.

ORGANIZATIONAL STRESS AND THE PROCESS OF CHANGE

From a multisystemic perspective, the institutional environment is pervaded by a set of common strains. Displaced workers come out of a troubled workplace that is undergoing a process of structural change and redirection of manufacturing efforts as a result of automation and competitive economic conditions. These workers, who are entering into a transitional phase, confront a job market which has itself become truncated. They encounter barriers when they seek employment within the same industry. Their experience is devalued because they symbolize the diminishing role of labor-intensive industry in a service economy. In the service industries, such as retail trade, the layoff is usually the result of mergers. The public sector institutions responsible for unemployment benefits and employment assistance purport to operate out of altruistic motives. However, these systems also devalue the intrinsic worth of displaced workers by disregarding their experience, prior economic status, and occupational identity. Displaced workers are thrust suddenly into a different role, which may be stigmatizing and downwardly mobile.

The current emphasis has been on public-private partnerships in the delivery of human services. This arrangement has brought together systems that have disparate core values. Private sector organizations, with their emphasis on profit and performance and on a clear distinction between labor and management, expect initiative and self-motivation as necessary employee attributes. Public sector organizations, emphasizing the altruistic and paternalistic role of government, even though ambivalently, expect their employees to comply with bureaucratic routine. The motive for public-private collaboration is essentially economic, namely, to reduce the extent of government spending on public problems and to redirect these funds to private sector concerns. The usual attitude of private sector employees towards their counterparts in the public sector with whom they interact in such collaborative efforts is that the latter are less capable, less motivated, wasteful of resources, and, overall, less professional. The public employees, likewise, regard their counterparts in the private sector as entrepreneurial, self-interested, insensitive, and rigid. They collude, however, in their mutual distancing and, at times, disdain for displaced workers whom they regard as dependent, less entitled, unrealistic in their economic expectations, and somehow responsible for their own predicament. This shared attitude of "victim blaming" reinforces the view of the displaced worker as a member of the "underclass."

The strain produced by this dissonance between staff in both of these systems interferes with program effectiveness. The pressures toward successful placement, upon which reimbursement for service is determined in the private sector, lead to preferential selection. The public sector organizations within this partnership experience similar pressures to produce statistical evidence of favorable outcome. The difference, however, is that unlike their counterparts in the private sector, the staff in these public sector organizations is less threatened by job loss as a result of poor-performance-based statistics.

The displaced worker becomes a pawn in this process of selecting only those individuals with attributes that are salient in the current job market. The more observant individual is aware of the situation, and this then becomes an additional stressor. This perception leads to a sense of distrust and, perhaps, alienation from the helping process. The behaviors that reflect this attitude are refusal to participate in organized efforts sponsored by formalized reemployment and job-training programs, thus reinforcing the views and beliefs of program staff regarding the unworthiness of these clients.

Mental health professionals, through consultation to these organizations, can focus on this dilemma. The triad of the public sector employee, the company representative, and the client becomes the subject of intensive exploration. By assisting staff in exploring their attitudes and beliefs towards the client, i.e., the displaced worker, that intrude upon the helping process, these service providers can improve their performance and achieve program goals. Gerald Caplan's (1970) concept of "theme interference" is particularly relevant in this context. Theme interference describes a process whereby the client is stereotyped and, as a result, the predicted outcome is negative. The service provider is unconsciously inhibited by the process of theme interference and the client is at a disadvantage because of this attribution. These stereotypes may pertain to the client's age, ethnicity, gender, occupational classification and, in even more general terms, the label of "being unemployed." The service provider will extend assistance only to those clients perceived as worthy. Since theme interference intrudes upon their predictive ability, the resulting frustration and anger limits their helping efforts. This process of selective perception and behavior with regard to client worthiness produces failure professionally, and also produces what has come to be called "burnout" among service providers.

The mental health professional can reduce the intrusiveness of theme interference by entering into a consultation relationship with service providers, albeit as a peer with a common concern for the client and the success of the program. By reflecting upon the problem areas that interfere with achieving successful placement outcomes, issues of ageism, sexism, racism, and elitism can be examined. As the group of service providers begin to recognize their common concerns, effective planning can be initiated. The consultant avoids confronting the stereotypes about clients, but rather focuses upon these negative attributions as obstacles to be overcome.

THE LABOR UNION REPRESENTATIVE AS CONSULTEE

The labor union representatives involved with displaced worker programs are frequently the community services representative, the benefits representative, the vice president, and, at times, the shop steward. During the entry stage, the mental health professional must develop linkages—i.e., establish ties—with the labor union leadership and members of the affected work force. These linkages must occur on several levels in order to assure acceptance within the affected system. The professional must be introduced to a representative of the target population, who may be from the company or the union. The purpose of this introduction is to become familiar with the circumstances of the closure.

The mental health professional needs to make a "quick" systems analysis of the affected work force, the work environment, and the industry. Retail stores, hospitals, and others in the service sector have work settings that are familiar to the mental health professional. A briefing about the nature of the work and composition of the work force, however, is essential for an understanding of less familiar work settings. These introductory efforts accomplish three objectives during the entry stage. The consultant becomes familiar with the organization of the work, and through these efforts indicates an interest in the consultee's situation and facilitates trust building. This process is essential to the success of the consultation because it reduces the distance between the professional and the representatives of the target population.

During the entry stage of the consultation, the professional becomes familiar with the environment, the scenario, and the key players. He or she gains system-level information with respect to relationships within the union, problem areas, and corporate culture at the workplace. The professional has the opportunity to provide information about her or his background to representatives of the target population. A sense of trust, therefore, emerges out of this initial process of familiarity and demystification. Another outcome is the opportunity to analyze and diagnose the structural issues involved with this particular work force. The consultant, therefore, enters with a model for intervening in a setting, even one that must be modified to fit the particular needs of the affected population.

Potential obstacles may arise in the consultant's interactions with the members of the labor union. Decision-making in these organizations routinely comes about through a committee structure. It is important, therefore, to understand that one will probably be meeting with a committee rather than an individual, because this tends to be the preferred mode of communication. It is equally important that one recognize and accommodate oneself to a negotiating style that derives from the process used during labor–management bargaining transactions and other union activities.

CASE

The initial planning process of the United Auto Workers-General Motors Southgate assembly plant closure involved leadership from the union local, the state Employment Development Department, and key members of the local union executive committee. The local president expressed the need for stress counseling services. A second meeting was scheduled so that representatives from the State of California Department of Mental Health, the local mental health center, and the union local could explore the need for direct services. At this meeting held at the union hall, union representatives expressed concerns about reported suicides, increased illness episodes, and other stress-related phenomena. This group of union leaders was multiethnic and included younger and older workers. They shared their concerns regarding stress-related problems but disagreed about the type of program best suited to the union members. The benefits representative stated that the members were going to need a great deal of help because of the layoff. The vice president stated that this effort would deplete union funds and added that "they expect too much." The local president then expressed his view that the "older group had nothing to worry about" because of the financial benefits that would come their way because of the union contract.

The theme interference that emerged during this meeting was the "we-they" theme reflected in ethnic stereotyping and ageist biases. The statement took the form of stereotypes by the older leader regarding the younger ethnic minority workers' dependent attitude with respect to the union's ability to find employment for them. The younger union official attributed blame to the older leader's poor negotiating of contracts that led to the plant closure. The mental health consultant steered the group back to the issue of common concern, namely, the welfare of the union family. The consultant was informed after the meeting that intergroup tensions based upon ethnic lines were taking place. These same themes reemerged during subsequent meetings with the union leadership, and the consultant always returned to common concerns of the work family. This case demonstrates how a consultant receives information, formally and informally, during the entry stage.

THE PUBLIC SECTOR REPRESENTATIVE AS CONSULTEE

The representatives from the public sector who are involved with displaced worker programs are usually middle management personnel within the state job agency, commonly referred to as the "unemployment office." These individuals are responsible for meeting with representatives of the union and the affected company during the pre-plant closure phase.

CASE

Supervisory personnel of the state employment department assigned to work with a large-scale industrial layoff met with the labor union representatives and the coordinator of mental health services for this project. The purpose of the meeting was to discuss the poor attendance at job-search workshops that the state agency had developed and were offering as a service. The major complaint expressed by the agency staff members was frustration over the clients' unwillingness to participate in these special efforts offered on their behalf. The issue of the displaced workers' attitude towards lower-paying job offers was presented as a source of irritation. A supervisor of employment services stated that "they have been overpaid for so long, and now they expect us to baby them . . . and nobody babies me." The theme interference is the perception of the displaced worker as acting inappropriately dependent and "like a spoiled child." One of the supervisors expressed her belief that these workers were already receiving preferential attention through the establishment of this special program. Informally, comments were made about the disparity between hourly wages paid to these auto workers and those earned by public employees.

The "spoiled child" theme created resistance among agency staff. It became apparent to the consultant that the job-search workshops were unpopular because the displaced workers perceived the staff members' hostility towards them. The consultant pointed out that the leader of the workshop might be experiencing a sense of rejection because of the poor attendance and encouraged more involvement with the union leadership. The purpose of this consultation was to reduce the image of passivity and dependency attributed to the union leadership. In practical terms, the conflict was reduced through increased union involvement with the state employment agency staff by assisting in mailing notices and co-signing announcements of upcoming job-search workshop sessions, as well as co-sponsoring these workshops and other job-search-related activities.

THE TRAINING AND PLACEMENT SERVICES REPRESENTATIVE AS CONSULTEE

The representatives from the training and placement institutions involved in these programs are usually middle management, such as program directors and others administering the delivery of services to displaced workers. Their role is frequently to acquire alternate sources of funds for their programs in a highly competitive vocational training market. A key stressor emerges from the demands for measurable performance of services. The term "performance-based contract," arising from federal and state mandates, places pressures on service providers. A typical contract requires that a participant be placed in a job for a minimum of 31 days before full compensation will be made to the service provider. This contractual arrangement, enforced by government funding agencies in recent years, often decreases the motivation to work with those at higher risk, such as older workers and less-educated and less-skilled persons. These individuals could well become "breakage" to the service providers, that is, a higher number of them will require more labor-intensive efforts in order to receive reimbursement. In terms of stress, the service providers experience high frustration and, in some cases, minimal reinforcement for their efforts. What one finds, then, is a system in which the providers of services and the recipients are functioning at less than optimal capacity.

CASE

The program manager and staff members of a prestigious high-technology corporate training center met with the mental health consultant to explore problems in recruiting and placing the displaced workers referred from public sector programs. The need for specialized stress counseling for these participants was also discussed. The program manager expressed pride in her organization's success in training and placing its students. She pointed out that *their* students were highly motivated, had good attendance, dressed appropriately, and were successful. She made the point that the school did not differentiate between the private students and those funded by the public sector. Her program assistant, however, quickly pointed out, "You can sure tell them apart." Another staff member added, "They're really more trouble to us, and don't live up to our high standards." The program manager indicated that it was the ideology, dictated by their corporate headquarters, that obligated them to accept *these* trainees. The company has a reputation of providing excellent training and is highly regarded by public sector funding agencies for its successful programs.

The dilemma for the training organization, then, was how to maintain high standards and still accommodate these "difficult" trainees. The consultant recognized the themes of differences and expectations, and encouraged the program staff to have the same expectations of "these" students—high performance standards and the appropriate attire they demanded of their regular students. The staff members were reluctant to make their usual demands upon the publicly funded program participants because of their unconscious biases. The primary concern of the training organization was the successful placement of their trainees in jobs. Their attitudes toward those funded by the public sector contributed to the failure of these students. The self-fulfilling expectation of the staff needed to be explored through the open exchange fostered by this consultation.

THE DISPLACED WORKER AS CONSULTEE

This consultation model is applicable to participants in these displaced worker settings. The consultant seeks to clarify the mutual objectives among the three components that comprise displaced worker programs, namely the client, the public sector employee and the employer. Displaced workers, as a client population, must perceive the helping efforts offered to them as being in their best interests in order to assure the success of these programs. These workers are experiencing loss and threats to their economic well-being and their sense of personal autonomy. Some lower-skilled workers, for example, express the recurring themes of bitterness and despair over their difficulty in moving beyond this phase in the process of dislocation. Many did not pursue educational opportunities and they have not progressed on an occupational track that allows for skill transferability. For many workers, there were legitimate obstacles, such as poverty, ethnicity, and inadequate schooling, and, for women in particular, socialized role expectations that limited their educational opportunities. Their experience in a lower-skilled occupation does not provide them with any advantage in the job market, since younger unskilled job applicants can replace them. These workers frequently express regrets about missed opportunities for training and advancement, and often blame themselves for their current situation of joblessness (Sennett & Cobb, 1972).

These same themes are expressed by semiskilled workers who see their upward mobility limited, perhaps jeopardized, by the lack of professional education. In fact, the origins of their dilemma may be similar to those of the unskilled workers. In attempting to rationalize their emotional reactions to being unemployed, they frequently introject the negative image to which they have ascribed and imputed to the chronically unemployed, the welfare recipient, and others who have been unsuccessful as wage-earners. This image of the "unacceptable self" is, perhaps, the major theme interference that the mental health professional must confront during consultation with displaced workers.

CASE

Paul was married, in his early fifties, and the sole wage-earner in his family; his grown children were out of the home. He was a semiskilled worker in the electronics industry and had advanced within the company for which he had worked for 27 years. The employees had been notified of the pending layoff and the anticipatory stress of the event was affecting his mood. He was eligible for early retirement at age 62 with a limited pension. Paul had mechanical skills and could have occupied himself, during this "time out," with projects in the home. His anxiety and depression, however, interfered with his ability to begin any of these projects, although he was aware of many that needed to be done. He expressed the feeling that he was "in the way," i.e., in the home during the day when his wife was accustomed to having the house to herself to do her chores or enjoy her privacy. The man appeared disheveled because of his need of a shave, although his attire was neat and appropriate. This industrial worker very much wanted and needed new employment, and harbored the hope that the old company would rehire him. He had been looking for other jobs and at the root of his depression was the fear that he was too old to be hired. His depression suggested longer-term issues, although his economic situation was realistically bleak.

It was apparent to the mental health consultant that Paul was at risk for developing a clinical depression resembling a post-traumatic stress disorder. Paul's immediate need was for a catalyst toward action. He was confronted with his self-imposed obstacles and offered job search assistance, since he was an experienced, competent, and respected person. His self-presentation, coming to the Re-Employment Center unshaven, discouraged the job placement staff from helping him. When confronted with the incongruity of his verbal expressions of motivation and his grubby appearance, he was able to see this disparity and to acknowledge his real wish that the old job would reappear.

The phrases that one frequently hears in this referential context are "I should have known . . . ," "I didn't listen to . . . ," "I wish I had . . . ," and other expressions of failed opportunities. Some other phrases heard among this group of workers include, "I had to marry and support a family," and "I had to take care of my kids," and other expressions of premature responsibility and economic necessity. Many displaced workers reflect upon their lack of motivation during their school-age years and their troubled family backgrounds that interfered with their striving for achievement, including the absence of role models.

The challenge to the mental health professional, when these themes emerge, is a complex one. There is a legitimate reality underlying this sense of frustration. In consulting with displaced workers, one needs to refrain from presenting false promises, validating negative self-images, or denying individuals' perceptions of their own past circumstances. The mental health professional also needs to be cautioned against attributing blame to these clients for their lack of achievement or attaching a characterological label to them. Professionals may tend to subscribe to a class-bound ideology based upon individualism and achievement. Therefore, when this theme emerges among clients, they may either reinforce the feelings of helplessness or deny the validity of their clients' reflections on their life situations.

DYNAMICS OF INDIVIDUAL CONSULTATION

The consultation interview is an in-depth assessment of the displaced worker's personal issues. The focus is exclusively on current status and work-related issues, as well as on potential obstacles, both objective and self-perceived. A formal assessment takes place during the process of individual consultation. The purpose of using psychometric instruments is for a quick diagnostic scan and for research and program evaluation. In some instances, however, one might choose to use vocational exploration instruments to help individuals further define their career goals.

The assessment measures used in our clinical work and research have included our own initial interview, the Profile of Mood States (POMS), the Brief Symptom Inventory (BSI), and a self-administered stress and coping questionnaire, based upon the Holmes-Rahe Life Events Scale, developed by the State of California Department of Mental Health. These measures provide the individual with feedback regarding stress level, coping strengths and weaknesses, and some personal recommendations regarding the need for more social support. Although we have not used these measures for diagnostic purposes, they indicate the presence of pathology. When a client presents with a severe emotional problem, referral information is provided and we adhere to sound clinical practice in making a referral in crisis situations.

CASE

Julie was a second-generation Asian-American in her late 40s who was laid off as a unit manager as a result of a company closure in the retail food industry in which she had worked for over 15 years. She was divorced and had recently separated from a longer-term relationship with her lover who lived with her. She had four grown children who appeared to be successfully employed. Julie's principal concern in reentering the job market centered upon the obsolescence of her business skills that she had developed during and after high school. She was very clear in her determination to avoid returning to the retail food industry because of the physical demands of that occupation, especially lifting and long periods of standing on her feet. She became anxious and pessimistic about the likelihood that the "system" would assist her in being retrained, in view of her age and job history. Julie reported herself to be a rebellious person who had departed from the traditional surroundings of her childhood by deliberately moving from an Asian-American neighborhood. She continued to defy family tradition through divorce and a longer-term nonmarital relationship with an Anglo lover.

All of this information emerged out of the individual consultation interview in an open, self-disclosing, and also assertive approach. Julie was highly motivated to change her vocational path in almost a defiant and independent manner. Her sources of emotional support included her children who were encouraging her independence. She was a physically active woman, with a high level of personal motivation. Her reaction to job loss was ambivalent in that she was making an adequate income and receiving excellent job benefits in work with minimal job satisfaction. Her life satisfaction was focused outside of the workplace. She regarded herself as a good worker, although she avoided customer contact. Her interpersonal style of being defensively abrasive seemed to be a deterrent to job counselors who perceived her as being a potential problem client.

The technique of the consultation interview is closely related to that of shorter-term therapies, such as crisis counseling, in the focus on the here-and-now coping skills and a rapid assessment of the need for therapeutic intervention. The mental health professional is clearly interested in determining to what extent a person's stress level is intruding upon the process of change. Family matters are touched upon as they pertain to job and work-related issues. The job history is discussed, particularly with reference to career and vocational limitations, as well as the client's educational background, including consideration of cognitive deficits and learning disabilities. Demographic factors, such as sex and age, are discussed, as are risk issues, such as concerns with health status and physical disabilities. Finally, the clinician reviews the client's previous personal crises to determine whether there is a history of severe stress disorders. The consultation process, from the client's perspective, enables the individual to bring up in the interview issues that he or she may resist talking about in group sessions. The interview gives the client a sense of both having an ally and being considered as an individual rather than as a member of a class of displaced workers.

5

Shutdown at Southgate: The Closing of a General Motors Assembly Plant

The case study presented in this chapter concerns post-layoff experiences of a group of displaced auto workers who participated in an industrial retraining, job placement, and counseling program in Los Angeles, California. Sponsored jointly by the United Auto Workers (UAW) union, General Motors (GM) Corporation, and the State of California, the program was designed to prevent or reduce the social, economic, and personal problems associated with longer-term unemployment. The Counseling Program for Displaced Workers was established at the GM/UAW/State of California Retraining and Reemployment Program's site at the Local 216 union hall in Southgate eight months after the GM assembly plant shut down there. The program staff provided counseling, prevention services, stress management, health promotion, technical assistance, and organized self-help groups for the displaced workers for the period of one year.

During the first month of the program's operation, clients sought help with financial problems, including confusion over benefits and delays in receiving unemployment insurance checks. Many had been experiencing family-related stresses as this was the first holiday season after the shutdown. Financial issues, such as accumulating debts, threats of foreclosure, and utility cutoffs, were frequently reported during this initial period of service. Shortly after this program began, rumors spread among workers about the possibility of a mass relocation to assembly plants in out-of-state locations.

Stress counseling program staff shared limited office facilities with state employment agency personnel at the union hall during the first months of the project. These arrangements enabled the staff to develop informal relationships with union officials, the displaced workers, and the state employment agency staff in this setting. Groups of jobless union members congregated to get information and to meet with co-workers. The workers were always aware of each other's help-seeking from the counselors because of the openness of the environment. Despite this lack of privacy, the setting of the union hall provided an informal and familiar environment in which professional and peer counseling could be provided. Individuals came in for help without prior appointments. The reemployment center, which was subsequently established by the state employment agency specifically for displaced GM workers, provided a more formal treatment setting. Private offices for program staff, coupled with less traffic and lingering of co-workers in the new setting, rendered individual help-seeking more confidential.

THE NEEDS ASSESSMENT

A survey questionnaire was designed to ascertain the needs of these workers as they returned to school to enter a new trade. The survey also probed their mood affect, morale, health status, social support, and expectations regarding their return to work. The questionnaire was pretested among six cohorts of workers, including those in retraining programs and those who sought direct placement for full-time employment. Displaced workers, representing 19 retraining programs (N = 304), were surveyed, and their responses were compared with those who sought only placement services (N = 223). The sample included a cross-section of participants at various stages of their training and job-search efforts. Women, who had entered training programs in such fields as electronic technology, refrigeration mechanics, clerical typing and office procedures, represented 5% of the sample.

In response to a question about problems that they were experiencing while participating in the intervention program, 55% of the trainees and 59% of the placement group indicated financial stress; 26% of the trainees reported family stress compared with 11% in the placement group; one-third of the trainees reported that they were having difficulties finding time to study at home and limited opportunities for leisure activities with their families compared with less than 10% of the placement group; and 18% of the trainees experienced transportation problems compared with 11% of those seeking job-placement services.

In response to a question on mood affect, trainees reported higher levels of worry (39%), nervousness (37%), anxiety (30%), depression (27%), and anger (20%), compared with the placement group's self-reported worry (22%), nervousness (29%), anxiety (20%), depression (15%), and anger (7%). Twenty-four percent of the trainees and 21% of the placement group reported feeling too old to undergo this occupational transition; and 20% of each group reported feeling good about the new undertaking.

Responses to a question on help seeking indicated that 24% of the trainees and 16% of the placement group wanted some form of individual counseling; 52% of the trainees wanted group counseling compared with 20% of the placement pool; 41% of the trainees expressed a need for other forms of help, such as tutoring and car pools, compared with 19% of the placement group.

When asked about their overall physical health over a three-month period, 15% of the trainees and 11% of the placement group self-reported poor health; 32% of the trainees and 27% of the placement group indicated fair health; 34% of the trainees and 41% of the placement group reported good health; and 19% of the trainees and 18% of the placement group reported excellent health. Although consistent between the two groups, these indicators of self-rated health status are disproportionate in comparison with a national sample of the United States population in which 5% of those sampled self-reported poor health, 13% fair health, 42% good health, and 40% excellent health (Ries, 1983).

When asked about their sense of confidence over the same time period, 20% of the trainees and 12% of the placement group reported that they had not felt confident; 47% of the trainees and 34% of the placement group felt confident sometimes; 19% of the trainees and 27% of the placement group felt confident often; 14% of the trainees and 27% of the placement group could not say or chose not to answer the question.

Two questions probed workers' perceived social support, particularly the exchange of helping resources within their social networks over a three-month period. In response to a question on help seeking, 52% of the trainees and 29% of the placement group indicated that they had asked a spouse, close friend, or relative to help them solve an unexpected problem; 37% of the trainees and 51% of the placement group had not sought such help; 11% of the trainees and 20% of the placement group could not say or chose not to answer the question.

When asked if they had helped or advised friends or relatives during that same period, 55% of the trainees and 40% of the placement group indicated that they had offered support; 32% of the trainees and 40% of the placement group had not done so; and 12% of the trainees and 18% of the placement group could not say or chose not to answer the question. Although trainees had mobilized the helping resources of their social networks to a greater extent relative to the placement group, the pattern of response indicates a client population that is hesitant in their help-seeking behavior and not confident enough in themselves to offer support to friends and peers.

When asked when they could expect to be working again, 15% of the trainees and 16% of the placement group stated either upon finishing training or within one month after training ended; 16% of the trainees and 7% of the placement group thought it would take longer than one month; 3% of the trainees and 2% of the placement group stated that they would not be able to find a job; 65% of the trainees and 63% of the placement group reported that they did not know when they would be working again; 2% of the trainees and 12% of the placement group chose not to answer the question. The overall pattern of response to this question is indicative of the uncertainty and conflicts that workers were experiencing when this survey took place, that is, in the weeks immediately following the announcement that the plant would be permanently closed and that workers would be asked to relocate to assembly plants in other parts of the country. The rumors that this event would occur had become reality.

SERVICES PROVIDED AND PATTERNS OF HELP SEEKING

Supportive services, including short-term crisis counseling and mutual support groups, were provided to approximately 2,000 workers. Seventy-six percent of those seeking services were self-referred, 22% were referred by union staff, and 2% of the referrals were initiated by California state personnel.

During the first months of the intervention program, the problems, for which help was sought, concerned basic needs: 33% of initial contacts involved requests for information about food; 33% were inquiries about other community resources, such as hospitals and clinics; 22% pertained to financial stresses; and 4% were inquiries regarding public assistance programs. Later in the year, clients sought help for more emotional problems: 6% in the areas of job search, relocation, and retraining stress; 1% for personal and emotional stress; 1% in marital and family problems; and only 5% in the alcohol and substance abuse area.

Over a one-year period, the clinical staff treated a total of 112 individual and family therapy clients on an ongoing basis. These statistics reflect a general trend regarding help seeking, perceived needs during times of unemployment, and the stigma attached to mental health services by members of industrial work forces.

The prevention efforts in mental health and health promotion, the support groups, and the stress management programs yielded the following pattern of participation: 407 workers were screened for hypertension at the union hall, at the reemployment center, and at the training institutions; 302 clients attended job search workshops where health promotion techniques were introduced along with training in effective job-seeking skills; 528 clients took part in mutual support groups held at the training institutions; 120 clients attended job clubs at the union hall, which offered self-help strategies for job seekers; and 126 clients participated in support groups dealing with the stress of relocation to other auto assembly plants.

STRESS COUNSELING

Stress counseling was provided to displaced auto workers on a short-term basis to prevent the development of more serious emotional problems associated with longer-term unemployment. As these workers were essentially normal individuals undergoing the transitional stress of sudden loss of work, retraining, and search for new employment, the intervention of a specially trained staff of professionals and peers at key points of crisis influenced the consequences of their situation. These interventions were designed to strengthen the workers' existing coping skills and self-esteem, to help them develop new and alternative ways of coping and problem-solving, and to help them to benefit from the resources provided for retraining and reemployment.

Individual clients were counseled on both an appointment and drop-in basis by a trained clinical social worker. The problems presented included family and marital problems, financial difficulties, excessive drinking, relocation stress, job training anxiety, loss of self-esteem, illnesses in the family, and so on. Most clients were seen on a short-term basis. Emergency services were available by telephone on a 24-hour basis. Crisis situations resulting from job-seeking and retraining stresses were the most frequent problems encountered. Informal contacts were available at the reemployment center, at the union hall, and at the training sites. These informal services usually reduced the displaced workers' levels of stress by providing a place to go for social contacts and by minimizing their sense of isolation and their hostility.

The goal of professional staff members was to provide direct assistance and to make referrals to the correct source. They helped clients with unemployment insurance problems by directing them to the proper channels, and thereby deflected frustration and anger. Many clients had problems because their benefits were delayed due to lost or misplaced records. Others needed assistance in filling out the necessary forms for unemployment extensions. Stress counselors also referred potential retirees to union representatives or General Motors staff members.

Clients had different expectations about counseling. Many assumed that the stress counselor would tell them what to do and provide quick solutions to complex problems. Others were skeptical about the counselors' ability to understand and provide meaningful assistance to them. At the onset of the program, many of the workers were uncomfortable about seeking help. Over time, however, referrals increased as workers' difficulties continued and stress services became more visible and less stigmatized. Outreach efforts by program staff helped workers to understand the counseling process, issues of client confidentiality, and personal, class, and cultural barriers that deterred them from seeking help. Clients were never told what to do, but were taught how to make their own choices and decisions, to weigh various alternatives, and to express their frustrations, fears, anger, ambivalence, and confusion. Counselors facilitated clients' development of useful coping strategies through information about existing resources, and by helping them to obtain assistance from various community agencies to meet their material needs.

PEER COUNSELING

Peer counselors were stationed at the union hall and provided information and referral for every kind of material problem: food distribution programs, utilities, rent and mortgage payments, and so on. The peer counselors were a major source of referrals to the clinical social worker for stress counseling services. Since many displaced workers were in need of food, a food distribution program was developed using government surplus commodities such as cheese and butter, as well as low-cost food packages distributed at the union hall. This program utilized many hours of volunteer time, provided a valuable service to the workers, and was a source of directed activity to many members who were neither working nor in training programs. The union hall also became the center of a free lunch program subsidized by federal funds.

Alcohol and substance abuse counseling was provided to eligible workers. Although both alcohol and substance abuse were recognized as serious problems by union officials, it was difficult to motivate the individual workers to avail themselves of counseling for this problem. The staff advocated for a number of individual clients in court cases involving driving under the influence. They also made referrals to Alcoholics Anonymous, Al-ANON, and public and private detoxification programs.

HEALTH-PROMOTION PROGRAMS

Workshops on prevention, health promotion, and stress management were offered along with mutual support groups, focused on transitional stresses and their effects. Among other subjects discussed were workers' lack of confidence in their ability to compete in the job market, complaints about, and frustration with, the retraining programs, and their preference for hands-on activities rather than didactic lectures. Workers frequently expressed anger and attributed blame for their current situation to the corporation, the union, the state agency, and the training programs.

The Human Relations Skills Training Program was a subsequent outreach effort that enabled trainees to discuss perceived obstacles, and reduced the risk of attrition in retraining programs. These self-help groups helped trainees to recognize their stress reactions and to cope more effectively by confronting problems early in their training, such as: (1) transition from the assembly line to work in a service industry; (2) interpersonal relations with training institution staff; (3) returning to a corporation auto assembly job requiring relocation to another city; and (4) developing specialized skills that would enable successful competing in the job market. From participation in the self-help groups at the training sites, the perceived stigma of utilizing individual counseling was also reduced. Staff members constantly reinforced the points that the program was for ordinary people facing difficult problems of daily life, and that helping workers with personal problems enhanced their focus on retraining and job-search efforts.

Stress counselors participated in job search workshops and job clubs that were held regularly at the union hall. The focus of these activities was on building self-esteem, assertion training, stress management, and worker motivation. These support groups facilitated the sharing of information regarding job-search strategies and helped develop self-presentation skills through role-playing. Mock job interviews provided a medium through which participants could ventilate their frustrations.

Health-promotion activities included dissemination of information regarding the prevention of stress-related illnesses. Blood-pressure screenings were offered in cooperation with public health facilities. Some 40% to 50% of the workers screened had elevated blood-pressure readings. These workers received follow-up phone calls by trained community health workers to refer them to appropriate health care providers in the community. Information was also provided concerning ongoing, free blood-pressure screenings held weekly at a community parks and recreation facility.

Staff members also offered a series of stress workshops to the staff of the state employment agency. A session on "Stress, Coping, and Social Support" introduced concepts of stress, psychosomatic illness, and coping through mobilization of social networks. Subsequent sessions focused on interpersonal relations in the workplace, coping with anger on the job, how to avoid burnout, and a self-help approach to stress reduction. These workshops helped agency staff to be more effective in dealings with displaced workers and contributed to the overall success of the retraining and job-placement effort.

COMMUNITY ORGANIZATION

Community-organization efforts of the project focused on developing a network of social service and mental health providers in Los Angeles County. Communitywide conferences were held for service providers concerning the special needs of displaced workers. Speakers from many sectors of the community, including mental health, labor, retraining programs, and state agencies, discussed intervention strategies and their effectiveness in serving the diverse needs of unemployed and displaced workers. The major themes of these conferences were: (1) linkages of corporations, labor, and government into a macro-network of a services in a period of structural economic change and deindustrialization; (2) overcoming the barriers to services among high-risk groups, including older, disabled, and educationally disadvantaged workers, and those experiencing discrimination based on age, sex, race, class, and culture; and (3) destigmatizing mental health services for this population through the development of care networks based on use of outreach to community institutions, peer influences, use of mutual support, and an empowerment perspective.

RELOCATION: A CRITICAL EVENT

A few months after the initiation of the stress counseling program, the company announced the possible relocation of

600 workers. Workers gathered in the union hall and at the reemployment center, and rumors developed even before the relocation notices were actually received and formal interviewing began. There was considerable concern about the uncertainties of relocation, relocation funds, strained family situations, and the potential disruption of retraining for new skills.

Three months after the counseling program had started, the interviews and screening of potential workers for relocation to the Oklahoma City plant began in the union hall. These events caused additional anxieties, fed by rumors surrounding the selection criteria for those who would be relocated, and whether previous work histories or medical histories would preclude transfer and completion of careers with the corporation. Rumor control was an important activity. Some of the rumors included: (1) the Southgate assembly plant would reopen; (2) those workers relocating to Oklahoma City or Shreveport, Louisiana would be laid off in 90 days; (3) the jointly run GM-Toyota Fremont facility in the San Francisco Bay area would not hire GM workers; (4) the Van Nuys GM assembly facility in the suburban Los Angeles area was closing down; and (5) various reports about the changes in benefit plans, including the Guaranteed Income Stream (GIS), pension, and other retirement benefits.

During these weeks, physical examinations were conducted, leading to another source of anxiety which was related to the fact that shortly after passing their physicals they would be reassigned to an out-of-state plant. The physical exam, therefore, was a concrete indication of this dreaded event. An informal "buddy" system developed, as those who were called for interviews and physicals contacted those close to them in seniority and on the shop floor in order to share information, compare notes, and offer support. Within a week or two following these physical exams, workers were receiving letters asking whether they would accept or reject offers of employment. Approximately eight days after this letter was mailed, telegrams were sent to a small number of workers requesting that they report for work at the Oklahoma City plant, approximately 1,400 miles away, on the following Monday at 6 a.m.

These events resulted in the following issues surrounding relocation: (1) a gradual building up of anxiety, nervousness, and worry; (2) self-destructive behaviors, including excessive drinking and substance abuse; (3) a lack of concern for personal appearance and public demeanor; (4) aggressive speech, including threats against those in authority at the reemployment center; (5) concerns regarding separation from spouses, threats of divorce, spousal depression, and spousal abuse; (6) concerns about financial insecurity, including house sales, the fate of the spouse's career, and debts related to relocation; (7) concerns about children finishing school and remaining in the home with only one parent, which might result in discipline problems, acting out, and depression; (8) the burden of maintaining two homes when the responsibility for one was already stressful; (9) the threat of initial "homelessness" upon arrival at the new job site; (10) the dilemma of training versus relocation, namely, how to make an informed decision regarding career prospects; and (11) concern over loss of California unemployment insurance if the Oklahoma job offer were refused.

Relocation issues that surfaced in the late winter following their layoff persisted throughout the spring and summer months. Unlike the Oklahoma relocation, however, subsequent recalls were on a more voluntary basis and appeared to be less stressful. Workers in retraining programs were able to obtain official postponements of recall in order to complete training. During this period, there was a large number of workers who were not taking advantage of the training opportunities offered to them and who were also not aware of the support services available to them. The reemployment center staff began a mail campaign in late summer following their layoff to reach these workers and, as a result of this effort, additional clients then availed themselves of stress counseling services. A substantial number of these clients sought assistance for the stresses associated with financial difficulties. Increasingly, they sought help for referrals to public entitlement programs, utilities shut-off assistance programs, dental clinics, and financial aid programs for college-age children. Many displaced workers were faced with the inability to pay their monthly rent or mortgage, to afford fuel for transportation, and to meet their monthly bills; some individuals, especially those with larger households, reported serious difficulty feeding their families. Many had to contend with the problems of delayed unemployment and benefit checks, making household budgeting a difficult task. The most common reactions to these conditions were frustration, anger, and feelings of helplessness.

An increasing number of individuals were having personal emotional problems, such as depression, thoughts of suicide, lowered self-esteem, and nervousness. For many, the pressures and demands of retraining, compounded by learning problems, led them to seek counseling. Similarly, the stress of looking for new employment in a tight economy, exacerbated by the upcoming cessation of unemployment benefits, led people to counseling. The most common reactions to these changes and uncertainties were fear, disillusionment, anger, and feelings of powerlessness and hopelessness. For other individuals, the psychological factors associated with being out of work affected their physical health. Clients reported substantial weight gain, sleeplessness, migraine headaches, stomach problems, and general fatigue.

There were an increasing number of family and marital problems. Many of these problems first surfaced when workers received letters from the corporation to report to work out-of-state. The prospect of relocation, possible family separation, or loss of partial income placed additional strains on family life. Some of the children of displaced auto workers showed a drop in performance at school and increased behavioral problems, and a few children exhibited illnesses associated with emotional stress. For workers who were not in training programs and who had low seniority, there was the cessation of unemployment insurance benefits, the depletion of long-held savings accounts, and the inability to rely on extended family for financial support. There were increasing requests for referrals to public entitlement programs. Families were faced with eviction, foreclosure, utility shut-offs, and drastic restrictions on their buying and spending, in addition to marital discord made worse by these financial difficulties. Many displaced auto

workers and their families were in a stalemate, both financially and emotionally. They had not begun to recoup their financial standing, since the worker had not gone back to work,
thereby continuing the uncertainty and confusion about the
future. As training programs ended, many workers still had
not secured new employment and were faced with two future
options: the difficult and frightening task of looking for work
in a new trade with only a few months of training or experience
behind them, or the disruptive but possibly more secure alternative of accepting or volunteering for a GM out-of-state relocation. Many workers completing their training programs reported that they would prefer to remain in California and find
jobs in their newly acquired trade. However, they also expressed a lack of confidence and a concern that they did not
have adequate training or sufficient experience to be hired in
new occupations. Relocation was a viable option for these retrained auto workers. For other displaced GM workers and their
families, out-of-state relocation was finally seen in a more
positive light as the best financial option available, because of
good wages, benefits, and union safeguards. The issue was
ultimately resolved for hundreds of families that did choose
to relocate. Family separation occurred, with many of the
spouses remaining in California, either on a shorter-term or
longer-term basis, while their husbands relocated. These wives
sought financial and emotional support at the union hall, and
they reported difficulty in maintaining two separate households, loneliness, worries about rearing and disciplining their
children alone, as well as fears of infidelity or permanent family
breakup.

With the ending of stress counseling services after one year,
clients were notified and referred to community agencies.
Although the social worker staff had advocated vigorously on
behalf of the workers with these agencies, very few union
members chose to take advantage of the services, because many
were uncomfortable approaching unfamiliar agencies with their
problems. As the intervention terminated, the problems that
surfaced were more serious in nature than in the earlier months

due to the extended period of unemployment and the continued uncertainty of reemployment and relocation.

CONCLUSION

The program model described in this case study was designed to provide ready accessibility for the displaced workers, to destigmatize the mental health image, and to encourage help-seeking behavior. This type of model was essential for the successful provision of mental health services to these displaced auto workers, as it was designed to take into consideration the needs of the individual, the family, the workplace, and the community. Although current research has indicated the health and mental health costs of unemployment, there has been a lag between this knowledge and the development of technical skills to provide effective programs. Mental health professionals have had difficulty modifying their programs for normal populations undergoing transitional stresses; personnel managers and vocational counselors frequently have lacked the skills to address the emotional needs of these populations. In addition, efforts have failed to attract participants, in part by unduly stigmatizing the clients, and ultimately not serving the needs of the community.

A systematic approach to program design would enable human service providers—including mental health professionals, vocational and rehabilitation counselors, personnel managers, labor organization and manpower agency staff—to collaboratively plan and implement effective stress reduction and crisis intervention programs for displaced workers, the chronically unemployed, and others affected by technological change. There is a need, too, for systems competency in implementing an effective, structured program to ameliorate the stress on workers during such transitions as plant closure, layoff, retraining, and employment in new occupations.

6

Competence and Empowerment: Prevention Approaches

JOB LOSS AND COMPETENCE

The individual who is competent at work tends also to be competent in personal relationships (Kohn, 1980). These multiple competencies (Gardner, 1983, 1984) are transferable to coping with both planned and unplanned job change. Those who are competent in their vocational skills anticipate timely reemployment because they have had more experience with success in their jobs and, prior to that, in their educational careers. Social competence, in a similar way, is an asset to both an individual's work and private life (White, 1979). Social skills make a person more attractive and, therefore, more employable.

More competent individuals tend to find other jobs before the plant closing. Some may actually leave the company before their layoff date, especially when the company does not place sanctions on them for early departure. Many companies establish a layoff date and provide severance pay to employees contingent on their remaining at their jobs until this date. This severance pay incentive serves as a "disincentive" to individuals with extensive longevity in the company, as well as those who have more pessimistic attitudes regarding the availability of new employment. There are others who, despite the economic in-

114

centive, will proceed to obtain new employment. These workers tend to be more individualistic, more assertive, and, therefore, unwilling to concede to the company's time line for termination. They are more competitive, as well, choosing to enter the labor market before their peers are laid off. The more competent employees are frequently assisted by the company in locating other jobs. These individuals also tend to have a stronger support system of friends and family that helps them to develop contacts with other employers. The more successful job seekers appear to be more flexible in their willingness to look for employment in other communities or geographic locations and seem to have less fear over the prospect of change.

It is really only the middle-class skilled workers who regard choice of job and choice of work as being within their control. Unskilled workers, by comparison, view having a job—any job that has stability, proximity to home, and with good working conditions and benefits—as sufficient for their sense of job satisfaction. These workers often do not have the same options for career decision making as the skilled worker. Constricted labor market conditions, skill obsolescence, and, at the individual level, personal characteristics are obstacles to successful transition. The labor market, with its shrinking opportunities for unskilled and semiskilled workers, has limited options. Increasingly, the companies that employ these workers have moved out of the urban regions in North America, choosing to relocate overseas where the cost of labor is lower. In the past, a semiskilled assembly worker, for example, could move from one company to another with little difficulty. There was very little need for conscious decision making since the labor market demands for these workers provided a plethora of jobs. These workers are now forced to confront and consciously resolve the problems of securing work in a constricted labor market. Without having had previous opportunities to develop their competencies in work skills and personal decision making, they are at high risk for permanent displacement from the job market.

There is, however, some degree of self-selection that occurs among these semiskilled and unskilled workers. There are those who attended school to improve themselves while they were working. These individuals, when laid off, view this transition as an opportunity to move into higher-level occupations, as they have developed a greater sense of personal worth along with their cognitive competencies. Their motivation to achieve (McClelland, 1961) can be directly related to this capacity to explore cognitive options prior to crisis situations, as in the case of workers who engage in continuing adult education during periods of stable employment. Many of the other semi-skilled or unskilled workers have had ungratifying educational experiences that may have thwarted their skill development. These individuals, unlike their achievement-motivated counterparts, may find themselves in serious economic danger because their skills have become obsolete.

Emotional competence has to do with the individual's capacity to adapt to change, to have a future orientation, and to recognize obstacles. The sense of emotional competence is, in part, a problem-solving process that requires active planning, rather than passively expecting that solutions will emerge. Finding a new job, then, requires that the individual integrate cognitive, social, occupational, and emotional competencies. When a person has deficits in any of these areas, this transition is less smoothly accomplished. A person with certain kinds of emotional problems, for example, who has been able to function in a stable work situation, may be at risk when faced with job loss. A steady job has served in many instances to anchor an individual whose emotional life is chaotic. When the stabilizing force that the job provides is threatened or removed, this person is thrown into a crisis. The resulting emotional insecurity and challenge of entering new and unfamiliar surroundings are often paralyzing.

PREVENTION OF ACUTE AND CHRONIC STRESS REACTIONS: TRANSITIONAL STRESS COUNSELING

The chronically mentally ill person, who is capable of functioning in a structured job situation sometimes with appropriate medication, will need assistance in effecting a job change. This form of support is not often readily available because the mental health system has only recently recognized the need for providing such services. There are physically and emotionally handicapped individuals who were hired by larger companies as a result of affirmative action programs. The therapist in a displaced worker program should be aware of the needs of this special population and link them back to the specialized resources in the community. These individuals are in both emotional and economic danger because of the restricted opportunities available to them. They tend to develop a strong bond to their place of employment, and indicate a sense of emotional loss and accompanying sadness about leaving what for them was a setting in which they were accepted and productive. This normalizing environment, when lost, places these individuals at high risk for emotional breakdown, and accompanying economic dependency and, perhaps, homelessness.

Individuals suffering from transitional stress conditions manifest symptoms similar to those found in post-traumatic stress disorders, as described in the DSM-III-R (American Psychiatric Association, 1987; Figley, 1988). These are such persistent symptoms of arousal as difficulty falling or staying asleep, irritability, difficulty concentrating, and some physiologic reactivity. Those experiencing transitional stress frequently report such generalized anxiety reactions as tiring easily, feeling on edge, excessive worry, and an increase or recurrence of such physical symptoms as headaches, weight loss or gain, heart palpitations, and insomnia. These reactions reflect the impact of job loss as an extreme stressor. Job loss may not meet the criteria presented by DSM-III-R for a post-traumatic event (i.e., " . . . outside the range of usual human experience . . . that would be markedly distressing to almost anyone" [p. 250]). However, for certain highly vulnerable individuals, job loss is an event that triggers a constellation of symptoms also found in anxiety disorders. The common element appears to be associated with reactions to separation and loss.

Many people display the range of behaviors and symptoms characteristic of anxiety disorders and post-traumatic stress reactions (Kreitler & Kreitler, 1988) when confronted with both the advent of job loss—namely, the termination notice—and the event itself. These responses are temporary for most individuals, and it is important for the therapist to recognize their transitional nature. It is essential that a client be informed that these are normal, predictable reactions to the stressor. Such knowledge in itself is stress-reducing and diminishes the threat to a person's emotional equilibrium. This normalizing perspective, combined with identifying an individual's coping mechanisms, is the initial phase involved in transitional stress counseling. This phase also involves validating the view that work and loss of work are central to an individual's functioning.

The second phase of the counseling intervention involves helping individuals to identify their effective coping skills so that they can draw upon them during this crisis.

The third phase requires the therapist to identify the particular hazard that is evoked by this crisis and that requires resolution—the perceived threat of change, separation anxieties, unresolved issues about education, and prior occupational failure. There are some individuals who experience extreme reactions to any threat to their economic livelihood. The intensity of their reaction to this perceived threat may be immobilizing and will heighten that person's emotional vulnerability.

The Crisis Interview

The crisis interview usually comes about at the request of the individual client, or on referral from the company, the union, or the reemployment center staff. The focus of the session is on the hazard, which is usually an external event within the family, illness, severe economic threat, or other situation that creates a state of disequilibrium in the individual. The crisis interview often serves as an initial intervention. When the displaced worker programs exist outside of a mental health center, we recommend that the worker receive crisis counseling.

The initial interview provides the clinician with a dynamic, diagnostic view of the client. Clinical interviewing skills assist the counselor in a rapid appraisal of the client's functioning and as a screening for those individuals who may need follow-up care. Clinical skills are required to recognize severe stress reactions, as these symptoms will be found in a predictable percentage of this population. It is clinically wise to inform the client of the source of these symptoms so that she or he can understand how the event of sudden job loss and the emergent stressors affect her or him. It is important to link the individual to appropriate services so that the longer-term effects of these symptoms will be reduced. This initial interview has to be both an evaluation and a feedback session so that clients may fully understand the impact of the event on their lives. Care must be taken, however, in introducing such feedback to clients, so that they do not become further traumatized by the clinical experience. Such iatrogenic reactions can occur when no attempt is made to provide closure in the form of a subsequent interview, referral to an ongoing group session within the program, or to appropriate community resources.

The introductory group session includes practical suggestions on how to cope with the impending transition by recognizing such symptoms as sleep disturbances, social irregularities, dietary, and mood changes. These topics are best framed in accessible language that participants will easily understand. They may even augment the facilitator's suggestions because the situation seems open and nonthreatening. Didactic materials regarding stress, prevention, and help-seeking can be embedded within the context of participants' experiential contributions to the session. This enables participants to view the group's primary function as a medium for them to share their personal comments with peers in a safe setting and to validate their definitions of the situation.

The facilitator, by sanctioning her or his personal response to the event, encourages members to speak before a group of their peers. These lesser skilled workers will often have little experience of engaging in this more formal group situation. Each individual presents a primary concern, permitting the facilitator to employ a problem-solving process that becomes useful to the group as a whole. All participants can, thereby, recognize their common concern—surviving sudden job loss—through a vicarious learning method, that of providing didactic information of universal import.

The facilitator can also reinforce the strengths of each participant as she or he relates progress made in individual problem-solving since the previous session. By observing an individual "working through," that is, the individual's struggle to consider alternative courses of action, the other participants are exposed to the range of options available to them. The facilitator promotes this process by structuring a didactic interchange between the participant and her- or himself. When the topic is the participant's future plans, for example, the facilitator requires that the individual be concrete in relating a "game plan." The theme that the facilitator develops didactically is that knowing what you plan to do reduces anxiety. This technique of cognitive appraisal enhances the individual's sense of empowerment. The "pink-collar" clerical workers, with whom this technique has been successful, relate easily to this mode of intervention. This method of integrating didactic and experiential content increases the members' involvement with the group process (Kolb, 1984), and decreases the likelihood of information overload.

"Mini-therapeutic transactions" occur within these dyadic interchanges, as participants bring their immediate concerns to the facilitator within the group. An older worker, for example, faced with premature retirement, questioned how she would adjust to life at home with a retired spouse, from both a financial and an interpersonal standpoint. The group facilitator explored the way in which she and her spouse had thus far considered this problem. It became apparent that there had been conflict in this long-standing marriage around issues of autonomy. This participant was concerned that she would lose the freedom she had as a working woman. She feared that she would become homebound and controlled by her spouse, as indeed her own mother had. The therapeutic transaction in this case consisted in helping this woman to recognize how she and her husband had, in fact, negotiated a relationship different from that of her parents. She was helped to focus on her feelings of loss in relation to the work family and to explore options of part-time work and volunteer activities that would maintain her sense of autonomy.

OBSTACLES TO EFFECTIVE INTERVENTIONS

Client Resistance

In order to be effective in either group or individual interventions with any client, both therapist and client need to agree upon a commonly perceived problem, a set of shared values, and other elements that permit communication to take place. The mental health professional, in a nontraditional setting such as a displaced worker program, does not have the protection that these shared attitudes provide. The displaced worker may behave like the unwilling client who is referred by the courts, the employee referred by the personnel department as a result of disciplinary action (for substance abuse) or the parent required to enter counseling as collateral to the child's treatment. In each of these instances, the client resents the forced compliance and distrusts the mental health professional whom she or he sees as an extension of and being in collusion with the authority structure, such as an ally of management or the union bureaucracy.

The mental health professional is presented, in such organized situations as retraining programs, as an adjunct who is there to "help the worker." The clients, for the most part, neither understand nor trust this proffered helping process. Their lack of belief and their distrust present a barrier to intervention that is difficult to overcome. The ways in which a client manifests these attitudes are (1) polite silence; (2) nervous agitation; (3) jesting and jocular hostile remarks, which many times conceal their distrust of the mental health professional. These attitudes may also mask the client's discomfort with being in a situation where feelings are discussed and where his or her privacy is threatened. Others may feel uneasy in a setting where they have difficulty understanding the language and the concepts, which they identify as outside their experience.

Additional obstacles emerge when the encounter with the worker occurs in the pre-layoff phase. These workers, who are on "extended notice," in this way remain in limbo because of the economic incentive to remain on the job. This could be seen as a time to explore job opportunities or consider options for career change while they still have economic security. These workers seem unable to make a commitment to new employment because of the uncertainty of their termination date. Many appear to be immobilized by this artificially extended period of separation. Many fantasize that the plant closure or layoff will not occur, that the company management will somehow change its plans and their job will be saved, or that the company will find them a new job and thereby rescue them from unemployment.

All of these wishes serve to inhibit these workers facing the reality of job loss and the need to take action. This inability to take action also occurs among those who know their termination date. Many of these individuals are inhibited by fears associated with change. For many, the impact of the event is not experienced as a reality until it actually occurs and they are, therefore, unable to make plans. For mental health professionals, the pre-layoff phase appears to be the ideal opportunity for the worker to plan for career change, skill upgrading, and learning interviewing and resume preparation skills. This transitional period, however, is not always perceived by workers as a "window of opportunity" and, therefore, it may not be maximized. Mental health professionals may have difficulty recognizing and accepting these attitudes, which run counter to their own point of view. This also applies to the frequently encountered difference in attitudes towards work and its meaning that are held by professionals and their blue-collar clients. Work and the job are essentially viewed as a way to meet this group of workers' survival needs. Individuals in occupations that have required extensive training and education may share a common view about work and career, since future planning was a necessary part of their success. Mental health professionals need to recognize that members of other occupational groups hold common views regarding the nature, conditions, and meaning of work. The intensity of feelings of powerlessness among unskilled and semiskilled workers, for example, is often related to their limited options for career advancement and choice.

Interventions with displaced workers and other unemployed are often predicated on the intention of motivating and otherwise assisting individuals through the transition of job loss to successful employment. Approaches to this transition, based on management values, career advancement strategies, personal ambition and rational planning, are frequently incongruent with the life view and situations of individuals who struggle to make ends meet. The heightened sensitivity of these individuals to the differences in their perceptions of the world and those of management and other professionals creates an atmosphere of distrust and hostility. These attitudes may be interpreted as resistance when the individuals in these workshops and groups are reluctant to present their views and are noticeably uncomfortable when others are self-disclosing. Many times, they mask their worry and concern and may appear to be unperturbed, since they have been socialized to conceal their feelings from those in authority. In settings where the group leader creates an atmosphere of trust and encourages individuals to express their points of view, a spokesperson will usually emerge within the group to serve as a catalyst for more active and expressive group process. This dynamic may lead to the group members' conscious awareness of their common concerns, and perhaps their capacity for mutual support and empowerment. There are, however, observable differences among groups composed of employees from nonorganized workplaces and those from union shops. The sense of empowerment derived from the language of negotiation is manifest in the expressiveness of those in unionized workplaces, since they have participated in a process that values workers' views. The views they express in relation to trade unionism at this time, however, reveal disillusionment and embitterment. Those in unorganized workplaces seem to be closely tied to the concept of the benevolent corporation, and likewise express their disillusionment with the betrayal of the patriarchy. The perception of either the company or the union as an agent that protects employees from the demands and risks of the labor market can paralyze an individual's personal sense of agency, or the capacity for action.

System Barriers

Advocates of mental health interventions for displaced workers have had difficulty in persuading influentials in human service systems to implement proactive prevention models for this population-at-risk. Agents within these systems often do not operate within a conceptual framework that incorporates preventive strategies. If these agents were to perceive the emotional stressors that accompany job loss as a problem, they would then be required to take action. Just as medical professionals who work with the terminally ill develop defense mechanisms to deal with loss, those working with displaced workers protect themselves against intense empathy with many of their clients' downward economic mobility and the resulting life consequences. Agents in these public systems often share a belief in individualism and economic achievement, and this ideology is reflected in both their personal decision-making and in the service delivery model. Since individual motivation for success is an ideological assumption of many human service programs, the emergent interventions for unemployed and economically marginal persons can be regarded as unnecessary for the "general good." These services, then, are viewed as solely for the "system failures," that is, for the least motivated clients who are the least likely to attain a positive outcome for the system and its agents.

The concept of "transitional stress" appears to be more acceptable to agents within human service systems. It is more congruent with their world view of structural economic change, its effect on the labor market, and the subsequent shift in employment patterns. They tend to view individuals whose job loss stems from plant closure due to technological displacement as more worthy of these special programs because the situation is "not their fault." When these same individuals, however, become outspoken in their demands for comparable wages and benefits, the human services providers retreat into a judgmental attitude. They believe that the clients should defer to the view of the benefactorial professional—the placement counselor, for example—and be graciously willing to accept that individual's determination, even it if results in lower wages and decreased job status. By accepting these public sector services, the participants in these programs may need to surrender their sense of autonomy. This is incremental as the client has sustained job loss, participates in a public program, and thereby experiences additional stigma, threats to self-esteem, and the accompanying emotional sequelae. Only after these insults to the client's sense of self-empowerment are acknowledged can the mental health service system facilitate more effective coping strategies for clients to overcome the reactions to these circumstances and succeed in reemployment.

The most difficult task for the mental health professional, initially, is to demonstrate that these interventions will enhance the success of retraining efforts. The mental health professional must build a trust relationship with administrative and program staff members. This is accomplished by becoming more knowledgeable about the structure of their system, and by keeping them informed of the nature and the limits of the mental health interventions. In this way, agency staff will understand that they share a common concern in providing the clients with skills that enable them to move successfully through the various stages of job loss and the transition leading to reemployment.

Many of the employment and training programs have "counseling" components. The term "counselor" has different definitions, including the job counselor and the vocational counselor in JTPA programs, the educational counselor at the training institution, and the placement counselor in the state job service office. It is easier to understand the counselor role within the context of job-search and placement activities than that of the "stress counselor," who uses this term as a way to deliberately avoid the therapist label. The clinician, therefore, risks losing her or his professional identity in trying to provide services in a nonthreatening manner (Becker & Strauss, 1960; Friedson, 1970).

By using a professional role definition that does not imply pathology, and therefore will not be rejected by the system and its clients, the clinician may experience a diminished sense of power. Without the clarity of identity, moreover, the professional must rely on such referential modes as curricula, teaching materials, and job descriptions to delineate and support both the role and its functions.

Others who identify themselves as counselors may feel threatened when stress counseling is a part of a displaced worker program. These individuals may regard this new type of counselor—the mental health professional—as a threat to their sense of competence and as invaders on their turf. Training in the behavioral sciences is part of the background of many who are employed in these human service jobs. They often became public sector employees, moreover, as a specialized career focus with an altruistic attitude and desire to be in a helping role. These employees tend to attribute to mental health professionals the frustrations emerging from their own career role, and they develop an ambivalent relationship with the clinician.

The quality of this relationship is often determined by prior experiences with mental health professionals, either stemming from their own treatment or their resistances to seeking treatment. They do, in fact, indicate by their statements a wish for help for themselves because of work-related stress. This is often shrouded in wit and indirect references. This style of interaction reflects a fundamental distrust of the attributed knowledge base of the outside mental health professional. The clinician, moreover, is regarded as intrusive and possibly usurping the desired part of their job, that is, the active listening and helper roles. They perceive the mental health professional's presence as a threat to the autonomy of their role as a helper. It is not unusual for staff in public systems to carry large case loads, leading to less available time to spend with a client, and thereby reducing job satisfaction. Specialized mental health services are often seen as paid for out of funds that could be used to reduce their work load. Staff members will often perceive the displaced worker and the longer-term unemployed person as a potential deviant and manipulator of public services and funds. They somehow think that mental health professionals are naive, easily conned by the client, and unable to "see through" their clients' motives. The consultant may be regarded as soft-hearted, a "do-gooder," and a "mark" for the clients' manipulations. These same staff members will admire the consultant's "savvy," particularly in handling the problem client whose behavior may be disturbing. This view is reinforced by their perceptions of the mental health system as possessing the knowledge of managing the difficult client who disrupts their system. Developing a trust relationship, therefore, between the mental health professional and the staff within these systems involves considerable effort and is best accomplished when the consultant is honest and straightforward.

It is important in planning and targeting interventions to recognize the role that the employee has played in the company over time. It is beneficial to learn, prior to intervention, the makeup of the work force, including work skills, cognitive competencies, language skills, and the duration of the employees' relationship with the company. The consultant will rarely know this prior to the first encounter with the clients themselves, as an outsider to the workplace and its corporate culture. This is particularly true for consultants in an intervention program associated with the negative events of layoff, shutdown, potential relocation, forced retirement, and the prospect of longer-term unemployment. Distrust, denial, and masking of feelings are operating in the workplace among management and staff during this crisis period. These organizational dynamics inhibit the free flow of communication about the company's plans, the management's true intentions, and the workers' attitudes towards the crisis situation. The following case illustrates these dynamics:

CASE: A PRE-PLANT CLOSING INTERVIEW

ZETA was an electronic manufacturing company relocating from the urban core of Los Angeles to a peripheral community north of San Diego. Another part of the operation was to move to Mexico in order to access a cheaper labor force and lower overhead costs. This move had been taking place over a three-year period, with management and technical personnel being offered an option to relocate. The formal announcement that layoffs would take place came approximately nine months prior to the plant closure. The actual layoffs took place in monthly phases, beginning six months prior to the shutdown. Hourly workers, including electronic assemblers, stock clerks, and maintenance personnel, were being phased out over a six-month period as it was the company's intention to maintain production during the phaseout period. These employees had been aware, for at least one year, that ZETA had plans to relocate out of the Los Angeles metropolitan area. They had chosen, however, to remain with the company until the plant shut down, because of the promise of severance pay and because the actual closing date was indefinite.

The initial contact with ZETA occurred at the workplace during a pre-layoff orientation conducted by the JTPA-funded agency coordinating placement and retraining services. The company personnel manager approached the stress counselors to express her concern about the well-being of the workers who had recently received layoff notices. She then initiated discussions with her supervisor, a company vice president, regarding the development of a pre-layoff stress counseling program. It became more evident during subsequent contacts with her that ZETA maintained a benevolent relationship with the workers, and that this policy extended to the availability of an employee assistance plan and a "protective" relationship developed by the personnel department. What had evolved from the discussions between the personnel manager and her supervisor was a four-session preventive intervention, with 15 participants in each group. Each group was to meet with the stress counselors for one month and the cycle was to be repeated every four weeks, for six months, until the plant was shut down.

The personnel department notified employees, in writing, of the proposed series of group interventions. The personnel manager assigned each worker to a group based on the work unit. (It is valuable to the success of these pre-plant closing interventions for the personnel department to assume responsibility for group formation and for scheduling of the sessions, as this reinforces the company's sanction for the activity.) It was important for the mental health professional to clearly identify and delineate his role as separate from that of the company and its management. ZETA's corporate personnel manager and this plant's personnel director were both present at the first sessions of this newly initiated series of groups. Their attendance inhibited many of the participants; others joked about their presence or made such comments as, " . . . and I don't care who hears this!" The personnel representatives chose not to attend subsequent sessions after discussing the matter with the counseling staff. They did, however, attend a special series of group sessions for a small group of language-limited Asian and Latino electronics assemblers.

The first series of group sessions were composed of shorter-term employees, who had worked for ZETA five-to-seven years, and included a greater representation of recently arrived immigrants. The later cohorts were composed of longer-term employees, who had been retained because of their mastery of a variety of skills. There were, however, a few longer-term employees in these earlier groups whose units were disbanded and who chose not to relocate. Compared with other displaced workers, who unequivocally directed their anger toward the company management, these employees were less willing to publicly express hostile feelings. The women with lower skills, many of Asian and Latino background, clearly lacked the English verbal skills and the confidence to express their feelings in the group. There were some women from these ethnic subcultural groups, however, who were more articulate and assertive, and this seemed to be related to their higher levels of skill and training. They expressed their self-confidence regarding their working lives in the future. The company had provided them opportunities to learn skills and to advance from the menial jobs for which they were originally hired to progressively more responsible work within the plant. When these women lose their jobs, however, they will confront the fact that their skills and their current status are not transferable in the competitive labor market.

This dim view of employment prospects was seldom expressed in the groups, and then only by strikingly articulate and insightful participants. It was clear that many group members were made visibly uncomfortable by this observation. The denial of concern about job loss during the pre-layoff period enabled them to remain seemingly less worried and more in control. A number of women, who were primary wage-earners for themselves or their families, were more direct in their expression of concern about their economic future. They did not, however, seem to blame the company for their situation.

There were a few women in higher-ranking positions at ZETA. They had climbed to the ranks of middle-management. Some of these women managers had chosen to leave the company rather than to relocate. They expressed a critical view of company policy during a special group session for management personnel. A few criticized the duplicity of the company regarding its actual relocation plans and the company's betrayal of its longer-term employees. These views were not expressed by the blue-collar workers in their groups, nor were they of immediate concern to the lesser-skilled women workers who had the day-to-day burden of routine labor in the factory, combined with the stresses of family life with which to contend.

The men who participated in the groups were the lesser-skilled maintenance, stockroom, and warehouse workers, who worked side-by-side with many of the women, and the more highly skilled machinists and technical workers. This multiethnic male work force ranged in age from the late twenties to early middle age. The men initially seemed self-assured, confident, and on top of things. They appeared to be looking forward to their jobs ending, collecting severance pay, and taking extended vacations before getting another job. After this initial display of bravado, however, these men began to disclose their apprehension and concerns for the future.

The younger men appeared to be apprehensive regarding the decision to risk entering a new occupation by means of classroom or on-the-job training. Several of these younger men had entered the employ of this company as unskilled workers and had received training and promotions over the years. They were angry with the company for what they perceived as poor management decisions that resulted in closing down the plant. The men who declined the offer to relocate did so because they distrusted the company management. They believed that they might again be at risk for layoff after having uprooted their personal lives. They insisted that the company's decision to relocate was based on the selfishness and lack of compassion of the top management.

The group-level interventions took place during the interval between the official notification of plant closure and the individual's 30-day notice of termination. To quote one participant, "I'm still feeling OK when I get home after a day at work; it's only when I think about having to return to *that place* the next day that I feel bad." Some individuals were having emotional trouble acknowledging the onset of the event. They still came to work each day and maintained their attendance and productivity as they always had. Most workers, in fact, complied with the company's demands for overtime, and with changes in work tasks and shifts as a result of the shrinking work force. The incentive for compliance with these changing conditions and the ensuing turbulence was the expectation of the severance package.

Any apprehension that these workers expressed was in regard to their economic survival, rather than to their feelings about loss and change. As workers reported their tasks within the company, there appeared to be an emphasis on more individualized forms of work and therefore less cooperative interpersonal relations on the job. Among the women, it was the single head of household and the older women who expressed a deeper level of concern over their situation. Among the men, the more expressive were the older workers and those acknowledging skill obsolescence.

Techniques derived from group therapy became very useful in enabling these workers to express feelings of being let down by their employer. The facilitators referred to the experience of others in their situation who had reported certain reactions to their job loss. They stated, "The people we worked with at Beta seemed pretty angry that the plant was being moved to another city. Do any of you feel the same way?" This form of referential learning freed participants by encouraging them to speak up and gave them some idea of an appropriate response. The group members were encouraged, thereby, to express their feelings about their situation. Finally, they were to understand and acknowledge that this expressiveness does have a therapeutic effect for them.

These workers had a great deal of difficulty in allowing themselves to express feelings about their situation. This may have been due to a variety of factors. First, their jobs demanded strict compliance and high productivity. Second, this was not an organized workplace, where the union leadership could influence their attitudes regarding loss and change. Third, this was a work force that had been "let down," one that previously had a sense of pride in working for this company, in the products that they manufactured, and in the promotional opportunities presented to them.

Many changes had taken place in management over the past few years while these employees remained working in the plant. The physical plant itself was sold to a neighboring manufacturing firm that leased it back to them. Even the employee cafeteria, for example, was taken over by a new company, so they no longer felt that it was "their cafeteria." There was a discontinuity in top management, so they could not blame a specific person or management team who was familiar to them for their situation.

All of this appeared to diffuse their emotional charge and had a numbing effect, leaving them feeling powerless and confused. In other layoffs, those about to lose their jobs have a common set of landmarks which become targets for their anger and also make the sense of loss clearer. The frustration of this work force was more difficult to work through. The common concerns of most displaced workers—namely, the fear for their economic security and their apprehension about future employment—were more difficult for this population to acknowledge and openly express. This may have been the result of the gradual erosion of what has been called their common "life world."

The social and behavioral science literature refers to this phenomenon as "mazeway disintegration" (Wallace, 1957), or the perception of disorganization and one's displacement from the familiar environment. In the ZETA case, this work force had been gradually uprooted by the concurrent events of the gradual deployment of company personnel and resources to the new location while they continued working as usual for the company. The turmoil that accompanied the announcement of the plant closure as well as the other changes in the work environment created a long period of stress and other anticipatory reactions to job loss. Organizational psychologists report that these anticipatory stress reactions also occur when reports of mergers and takeovers of companies are rumored in the workplace. Studies of disaster management on the effects of early warning of earthquakes, flooding, and other natural events suggest a similar phenomenon. Common to all of these events is a paradoxical reaction: denial that the event will occur even when presented with evidence of its likelihood, and anticipatory anxiety concerning coping with its effects. This is an example of the phenomenon of cognitive dissonance (Festinger, 1957), where persons find themselves doing things that do not fit with what they know to be the case.

The workers at ZETA presented a facade characterized by a sense of calm and distance, even within the group, in order to adapt to this dilemma. They were masking their affect and presenting a "cool" demeanor (Goffman, 1967). This masking enabled these workers to "hold it together," that is, to maintain their work role identity (Hochschild, 1983) so they could continue to perform their jobs each day. They had to learn to suppress their resentment, inhibit their anger, control their aggression, and comply with the conditions of production in order to remain functional at work. Such compliance assured them of receiving their benefit package, promised by the company, on their termination date. The ambiguity conveyed to them by management, who in reality were uncertain when the plant would close, contributed to their stress. What characterized this plant closure and contributed to the workers' anger was the fact that this was a profitable enterprise with an expanding market for its products, and that the decision to move did not take into account the value of a loyal work force. The sense of powerlessness, engendered by the preferential treatment of select managerial and supervisory personnel, was expressed by a few of the more sophisticated and outspoken veteran employees. When these attitudes were expressed by a minority of the workers, others were enabled to disclose their feelings of abandonment.

EXAMPLE OF JOB LOSS IN A COMPANY OF LONGER-TERM WORKERS

The closing down of the southwest regional catalog sales division of a major national retail firm resulted in the termination of over 100 employees, many of them longer-term employees. The Brand Corporation had provided out-placement services to their management personnel, referred to as "checklist" employees; the hourly workers, however, had not been offered comparable services. Brand had permitted the state employment agency to provide job search workshops and the JTPA-funded coordinating agency to provide training and employment services to this latter group.

It was during the orientation of hourly workers on training and employment options that the assistant director of personnel met with the mental health consultants. He indicated his interest in the counseling program, but claimed to lack the authority to negotiate these services. The coordinating agency, when negotiating entry, met with a good deal of resistance from the personnel director. It came as a surprise, therefore, to the counseling staff that their services were sought by this company. An executive secretary of a unit that was being phased out was assigned a leadership role in organizing single-session workshops for approximately 100 employees, in groups of 15 participants. These workshop sessions were held in a comfortable conference room of the 60-year-old Art Deco building, which was the flagship of the company's southwest regional operations.

These longer-term employees, who were being terminated due to corporate restructuring, regarded the company as a benevolent provider of excellent benefits, profit sharing, job security, and opportunities for personal advancement. Many of the women, in particular, had begun their work lives as older teenagers obtaining their first real jobs at Brand, and many had continued to work there from 12 to 35 years. Included in this group were a smaller number of employees who were regarded as part-time workers, although working the equivalent of a full-time work week. They were in this temporary status, without benefits, for up to seven years, and at the point of layoff were not eligible for retirement benefits or severance pay.

This work force was primarily Latino women. The few Anglo women in the group were the longest-term employees in supervisory positions. There were a small number of Black and Middle-Eastern employees representing a variety of work roles. This multiethnic group of workers performed a range of clerical work routines, including data entry, inventory, packaging, bookkeeping, and ordering. The supervisors in the group had progressed up the career ladder within these work units. The few men represented in these groups had worked for Brand for many years as merchandise managers and buyers. These men discussed the option of relocating to Chicago, although it was never made too clear whether that option actually existed.

There was little group sanction to express strong disapproval of the company. Brand had provided these employees with security and advancement opportunities over a long period of time, and a strong sense of identification as Brand employees. Their anger, if it existed, was softened by the company's generosity. These employees' collective denial process, however, was challenged by the part-time employees and a few other individuals. They pointed to the deception involved in their meetings with management where they were assured, up to two weeks before layoff, that no layoffs were planned. There had always been the threat, however, over the previous five years, of discontinuation of their catalog sales division. This threat had been reinforced more recently by the shutdown of the northwest regional distribution center in Seattle.

These stress group sessions were held in an atmosphere of farewell parties taking place, during the last week of work. Many of the longest-term employees expressed disappointment and regret that they were forced into early retirement. Some, however, seemed to have made contingency plans, and some

were looking forward to time at home after many years of continuous employment. They were anticipating the opportunity
to spend time with their families, including their grandchildren,
and, in many instances, with retired spouses. A few of the older
women, in particular, expressed some apprehension about having more time at home because of problematic family situations
or, in some instances, financial constraints since they were just
short of retirement age. These older workers also expressed
worry over the possibilities of finding new jobs.

Those workers in their middle years facing this transition
expressed the greatest concern over the transferability of their
skills. Very few of these employees verbalized immediate financial concerns, perhaps because of the availability of severance
pay and anticipated unemployment insurance benefits. This
group of mostly married women was unwilling to talk about
financial worries. Many of the women with younger children
looked forward to a summer at home with the kids and were
clearly putting off future work plans.

At least one participant in each group, usually a middle-aged
worker, would bring up the issue of loss of the work family.
This enabled others in the group to talk about sadness regarding separation from co-workers of many years. Since most of
the workers met with the mental health consultants only one
time, the intimacy and trust necessary for the disclosure of emotional reactions were not present. Many participants, however,
formed in clusters around the group leaders after each session
to share their more personal concerns, as well as to express their
appreciation for the opportunities to talk in the group. All
employees attending these initial sessions were offered a follow-
up group, away from Brand, after their termination date. Only
a handful of them returned for this session after the layoff.

A second group of Brand warehouse workers were the second target group for intervention. They were semiskilled and
unskilled warehouse workers who enjoyed the same benefits
and security of working with this company. They regarded finding other work as a fairly simple matter, since their tasks, including picking parts, filling orders, and working with heavy
equipment, required minimal technical skills. They saw no
problems, therefore, in transferring to a similar retail or whole-
sale distribution center because their skills were so unspecialized.

These warehouse employees, like other lesser-skilled work-ers, appeared to derive their job satisfaction from wages and benefits, and not from the work itself. Their stresses, therefore, were economically rooted, age-related, and less related to skill obsolescence and longer-term career goals. Their reactions to job loss were buffered by severance pay and by the company's offer of jobs in other locations within the region, albeit with lower seniority and pay. They looked forward to the money they would receive upon termination, and the job offers made prior to their leaving the company gave them a false sense of their salience in the labor market. These blue-collar workers, unlike their pink- and white-collar colleagues, displayed less pride in their work and seemed to have a shortsighted view of a work future. This lack of future orientation and identification with a skill or the sense of craftsmanship often results in less ego involvement around termination from a specific workplace. Some individuals, however, felt worried about being without a job and experienced a sense of having less of a competitive advantage in the labor market, even though they did not derive gratification from their work. Their affective posture appeared to mask these feelings, perhaps serving to protect their pride before a group of their peers. This masking took the form of denial that anything was wrong or that they were bothered by the impending event in any way. The effect of the stress may have been more internalized, since these workers concealed their feelings, and may have presented in the form of increased physical symptoms and more use of alcohol and drugs to sup-press feelings and emotional confusion.

In a group situation, these employees were restless, bois-terous, demonstrated a lack of concentration, and constantly challenged the group leaders. The male participants, specific-ally, may have displaced their anger towards management onto the group leaders. Their resistance to active participation in the group process may have indicated distrust of the group's pur-pose and the leaders' intentions, embarrassment about self-disclosure, and general lack of familiarity with this method of communication. The clinician needs to be cognizant of the negative feelings evoked by these behaviors, including avoiding engaging in a power struggle with participants, given their ex-ternalized negative attitudes. The group leader may reveal disapproval and react to their challenging behavior by becoming critical, rejecting, and thereby losing control. The attitudes and values of the participants may also challenge the belief system of the highly educated, career- and future-oriented attitudes of the professional. All of these reactions are indicative of negative transference.

These Brand employees often attended the groups, held during company time, to escape the drudgery of the work routine. It was unrealistic to expect intrinsically motivated interest to manifest in these groups. The challenge to the group leader, therefore, was to engage participants on a level that was relevant to them. Any intervention would have been rejected, if its primary purpose was seen as dealing with problem behavior, abnormal reactions, or mental disorders. Even the term "stress group" connotes maladaptation and, therefore, evokes greater resistance and stigma to participants. How the group leader relates to the workers at the onset, through trust-building and mutual respect, influences the course of the intervention.

There appeared to be four principal ways in which participants in both target groups expressed anxious reactions to the strain of impending job loss. Expressions of blaming were often the first indicators of stress. These took the form of self-blame or attribution towards others in the workplace, such as the foreman or manager, and decision-makers in the more remote corporate headquarters. Some individuals became preoccupied and almost obsessed with the theme of blame, as projected upon powerful others who controlled their fate. The resulting sense of powerlessness, reinforced by peer interactions, did seem to discharge anger. Self-blame, however, took the form of self-recrimination, and this would often result in feelings of diminished self-worth. These attitudes may have appeared as a preoccupation and an inhibitor of future-oriented actions. The blaming stance may, in fact, have been a delaying strategy that concealed fear of the future.

Verbal and nonverbal expressions of sadness were a second indicator of strain. The workers particularly voiced their regrets about losing the daily contact with their co-workers, with whom they had shared long-term life experiences. These feelings of separation and loss referred specifically to fellow workers, and rarely to the work itself or to the workplace. Sadness expressed by the older workers referred to the permanent loss of a work life. Sadness was often expressed among the other workers in humor, joking behavior, and paradoxical remarks concerning loss and transiency. Such remarks as "Not to have to see your ugly face every day," or "Gosh, who am I going to pick on now?" revealed the discomfort these workers might have been feeling in expressing their sadness to each other.

Abstracted confusion and vagueness in affect in regard to future employment plans were a third trouble sign. Some individuals shrugged off having to think about the actions ahead of them in planning and looking for a new job. This may have been masking the fear of facing their economic reality, and may also have been protecting the ego from others perceiving their vulnerability. This facade can be misleading, as it often conceals the individual's need for direction.

The workers' sense of ambiguity and uncertainty were a fourth indicator of stress. Although those facing job loss said they must work and needed to find new employment, perhaps even desiring new skills, they were confused by the requisite steps and seemed to be unable to process the information presented to them. This may have been a cognitive problem caused by emotional blocking, since anxiety will often block the information-receptive processes. Clinicians and others, however, who interact with those facing sudden job loss may falsely perceive them as unmotivated and disinterested.

DEMORALIZATION AND EMPOWERMENT

The process of demoralization has its origins in workers' declining gratification with their jobs. The worker's dissatisfaction emerges from such factors as the routinized work process, "traditional" management styles, and the absence of intrinsic rewards from job performance. This set of experiences transfers into a sense of demoralization that emerges when a worker must make a decision regarding future options. Preventive interventions must take these issues into account in order to approach the problems that the demoralized and poorly motivated client appears to present. This lack of enthusiasm that many clients present for planning their next steps after a layoff needs to be viewed within the context of their prior experiences at work. When work is solely to meet economic survival needs, one job is the same as another. The process of "de-skilling," or the limiting of an individual's talents and competencies through mechanized, routinized work functions, lowers an individual's self-esteem, pride in achievement, and sense of self-empowerment (Lerner, 1986). Skill obsolescence, for a person whose work task has become obsolete, is a particular hazard since that individual may have an underdeveloped work identity. The resulting lack of ambition and motivation attached to skill competencies and lack of pride in personal accomplishment inhibits the individual's ability to maximize the opportunities available to her or him during the layoff transition.

The roots of these attitudes go back to early socialization and experiences in the educational system. Assisting these individuals requires techniques that will foster both an increased self-esteem and a new sense of empowerment. The process of developing self-empowerment is twofold. First, the displaced worker must become aware of the impact of workplace demoralization on the ability to make decisions, cope with stress, and become achievement-motivated. Second, the individual must begin to recognize the stressors in the workplace that perpetuate this sense of demoralization, with its resulting low self-esteem, diminished achievement motivation, and feelings of helplessness. Self-empowerment results, for example, when individuals who have shared concerns form a mutual support group. Such common concerns as job loss and skill obsolescence bring individuals together who are in crisis and in need of support as a helping force. These groups allow participants to discuss perceived obstacles to training and job loss, to recognize stress reactions, and to cope more effectively early in the transition period. Mutual support groups are particularly effective during the pre-layoff phase, the period immediately following job loss, and while enrolled in basic skills and retraining programs. The consultant can be a catalyst to a change process, like the mutual support group, keeping in mind that there are biases implicit in the organizational cultures of mental health and other professionals that can serve as barriers to change. These include equating the individual's apparent lack of motivation, loss of job, and skill limitations with that person's intrinsic worth.

EARLY INTERVENTION AND PREVENTIVE STRATEGIES

The program model developed by the authors involves several levels of intervention with displaced workers, their families, their employers, the public and private sector employees that serve them, and the community-at-large. Primary-level interventions are designed to furnish employers, public agencies, and the community with mental health education to inform them about the normal reactions to the threat of layoff and to advise them about coping strategies that will lessen the psychological impact of this loss. The purpose of conveying this information to the public is to increase its awareness of expected and predictable stress reactions induced by the crisis. By increasing the level of community understanding of the circumstances surrounding mass layoffs and worker dislocation, the stigma associated with job loss can be diminished. The self-stigmatizing associated with job loss has a negative effect on psychological functioning, so that community education focused on lowering attribution of blame and building the sense of self-empowerment is a primary goal of prevention programs.

A secondary level of clinical intervention is programs provided during the pre-layoff and early post-layoff periods. These efforts bring together individuals experiencing a common event in order to prepare them for this change in their lives and to assist them in making the transition. This goal is accomplished by helping the workers express their feelings about job loss, and ventilate their anger and sadness in a supportive environment. These techniques are similar to the "critical incident debriefing" method (Mitchell, 1983, 1985) that has been developed to lessen the vulnerability to stress reactions among emergency service workers and disaster victims.

Secondary-level interventions include case finding and referral for individuals who require formal mental health treatment. Individuals are often suffering the symptoms of acute stress, and specialized skills are needed to provide treatment to this population with the understanding that their problems are transitional, situationally induced, and linked to the job loss.

Help and advice about personal problems are sought from the group leaders by the displaced worker, within the context of these secondary-prevention program activities. These persons may have difficulty expressing themselves in a group setting and will seek out the therapist for private time. There are times when the nature of an individual's problems demands this privacy. For many of these individuals, contact with a mental health professional is a new experience, and problems that had been latent are elicited, often unexpectedly, by this group experience. The therapist needs to be available, supportive, and informative in these contacts.

There are those individuals who have had prior contact with mental health professionals and who seek out the therapist and want to talk about past and current problems. Their motives include the desire to inform the therapist of their "sophistication" and experience with mental health language and techniques, their personal vulnerability, or a problem in their family situation. These individuals will sometimes seek referral information. There are also rare occasions when the therapist will be required to intervene in an emergency situation in which the client is at risk for suicide or other extreme self-destructive acts. Paradoxically, company personnel managers and public sector manpower program staff perceive the therapist most clearly in this emergency intervention role. This may reflect their own lack of understanding of mental health prevention strategies and also their own sense of panic and inadequacy in coping with the anger and depression they view among the displaced workers.

A tertiary level of intervention involves individuals who fall within clinical diagnostic categories and whose life situations are made more difficult by job loss. Clinicians need to recognize the traumatic impact of these events and the circumstances surrounding them in order to incorporate this knowledge into their treatment efforts. They should be aware that job loss increases the individual's vulnerability and also threatens a person's treatment progress. On a practical level, this threat to an individual's economic well-being frequently includes the loss of medical benefits, which may threaten his ability to remain in treatment during this life crisis. Therefore, job loss, as a traumatic life event, cannot be ignored by clinicians because of its potency on the functioning of an individual.

7

Clinical Perspectives on Displaced Workers

JOB LOSS AS AN INDIVIDUAL CRISIS

An individual's sense of personal identity and self-worth is attached to the job itself and often to the workplace. That person's sense of integrity also becomes threatened when she or he is stripped of these anchors and is faced with the humiliating, and often depersonalizing, set of experiences associated with sudden job loss. These include receiving an impersonal discharge notice, standing in line to register for unemployment insurance benefits, and seeing oneself as a member of that stigmatized segment of society labeled "the unemployed." Such experiences can be especially demoralizing for the person who has a long, consistent work history and strong identification as a competent wage-earner.

The requirements of public entitlement programs reduce all applicants to a common level. This leveling of workers from all skills categories to a universal state of powerlessness and dependence creates frustration, anger, and humiliation. The attitudes of state job service employees towards the client are frequently hostile, suspicious, and unsympathetic. Their interactions can be characterized as patronizing and often rude. The newly displaced worker entering the unemployment line is confronted, for example, with a rationalized bureaucratic process, that of "regulating the unemployed." This includes maintaining social distance and rigidly enforcing the rules governing the disbursement of unemployment benefits.

The tasks of those managing the cases of the unemployed are to oversee, monitor, and control the legitimacy of their claims. The regulations require that the recipient of unemployment benefits actively conduct a job search and document these efforts. The newly unemployed person is often embarrassed by his or her failure to secure a job during the initial job search, and is angered by the distrusting attitudes presented by the enforcers. As middle-class workers may share the view of the unemployed as unworthy, lazy, and exploitative of public benefits, job loss creates a sense of alienation that increases the negative self-image and self-blame and ultimately damages morale.

The individual facing such depersonalizing events will often develop a new set of defensive strategies to cope with the resulting insults to the psyche. The defensive structure required to buffer these experiences can emerge from the person's adaptive capacity and self-concept. The therapist needs to help the displaced worker to identify these self-defeating attitudes so that the experience of job loss is not allowed to be absorbed by the individual as a psychologically injurious event. The displaced worker needs to perceive and understand job loss as an economic event and not as a personal failure. Clinical attempts to foster conscious and critical understanding of job loss minimize the development of such defensive responses. This process of awareness can both increase a person's resilience and protect the vulnerable individual from the hazards that may result from the event.

"Being out of work," as compared with being "unemployed," is a temporary status. Those who have been "unemployed" for an extended period to time, perhaps a year or two, often hold a self-image that has been socially constructed, ascribed, and reinforced through an institutional career sanctioned through public institutions (Piven & Cloward, 1971). There are major differences, then, between the nonworking person of transitional status and the more chronic unemployed person. The person in transition identifies her- or himself as competent and productive. That person's identity is closely attached to the most recent or longest-held job. She or he regards her- or himself as part of a work force, her or his unemployed status as temporary, her or his skills as marketable, with opportunities for new employment. The more chronic unemployed person, by contrast, may develop a sense of resignation, despair, disillusionment, loss of identification with the work role, with a concomitant loss of status.

THE DISPLACED WOMAN WORKER

Older women have difficulties finding new jobs, particularly if their job experience is limited to one or two prior tasks and/or work sites. These women must confront such issues as the transferability of their skills, ageism, their perceptions and fears of forced change, the reality of their physical limitations, and the demands of the new job. If a woman has only a single skill, then her chances of reemployment are limited, particularly if her attitudinal set is rigid or inflexible regarding the type of task or workplace and her perceived skill transferability.

In one situation, women who had been displaced from a large retail chain would only regard future employment possibilities within other retail trade settings. This set of attitudes may be explained partially as a result of their limited repertoire of skills, and partially because of low ambition. Although many of these women had been employed for a number of years, they did not regard themselves as having careers. Work outside the home evolved primarily out of a necessity to complement the family income, to be self-supporting, or to become the primary wage-earner following the loss of the spouse's income, either through disability, divorce, or death. The home, the family, and the social interactions at the workplace were their primary sources of gratification.

Sudden job loss at midlife shook them into an awareness of their lack of either education or financial security. They were accustomed to being wage-earners; but, they had been socialized to a different role, that of homemakers, dependent upon financial support from their husbands and with primary responsibility for the children. These women did not regard their work as a vocation or "calling," where the task is a source of gratification. Rather, they viewed it as a temporary pursuit with no expectation of personal gratification. They had derived, however, as a "fringe benefit," a form of pleasure that was serendipitous to the work itself, namely, association with co-workers, socializing with customers, or identifying with a prestigious company. Coupled with the loss of these sources of gratification, their age, obsolete or underdeveloped skills, and expectations of high pay were disadvantageous in the labor market. These women were faced with the reality of needing a job and the recognition that working is an intrinsic necessity.

Their belief that they did not "need to work" was an illusion both for themselves and for other working-class women. Women in lower income families have for many generations been working outside the home in fields, in factories, and in family-run businesses. It is often the social and physical distance between the home and the workplace, however, that distorts this perception of women and their work. Many women in such jobs as sales, assembly work, and service industries prefer working closer to their home, and will seek work only in proximate locations. The loss of the job, therefore, creates a major disruption since newer companies are tending to relocate in industrial parks and regional malls, which are located outside of more familiar residential areas. Job loss as a life event, then, includes a sense of "mazeway disorientation," a distorted spatial perception brought about by the threat of relinquishing the security of the familiar environment, no less entering a new work setting.

It may well be that women with both limited education and job skills have a sense of self that leads to a narrower perception of safe territorial boundaries. Working closer to home affords them easier access to the workplace and availability to their children and families. Their social world remains moderately unchanged by the fact that they go to work each day. Despite the fact that they are working outside the home, their sense of the world does not seem to expand. This may serve the function of preventing the individual from "outgrowing" the boundaries established by the family.

This "miniaturization" of the social world serves to restrict economic opportunities, a situation that is not limited to women, but is more typical of them. Men, by contrast, have always been encouraged to adjust their behavior to the changing demands of the labor market, that is, leaving home and neighborhood to seek work, commuting lengthy distances, and migrating to areas remote from family. Women have accommodated themselves, until recently, to the needs of their families (Young & Willmott, 1973). Underlying this behavior is an assumption that women remain closer to the home and are the protectors of the home and children in the men's absence. This may be why women have traditionally supplemented the family income through such home-based activities as laundry, childcare, sewing, and so forth. In this way, the women were able to remain within the private world of the family. Their family worlds were the primary source of their self-definition, providing a close-knit network of relationships that was, for them, a deeper source of gratification than any job outside the home. Their emergent sense of self was based, therefore, upon an ethos of domestic responsibilities and caring for dependent children (Gilligan, 1982).

It is not uncommon among working-class women to hear them assert that they are not feminists (Rubin, 1976). These assertions, paradoxically, are often heard from women in such nontraditional occupations as carpentry and forklift operation. Many of these women are employed in a male-dominated occupation because of the breakdown in the gender-based segregation of job tasks. Their social attitudes, however, do not reflect the changes attributed to the women's movement, as they have not incorporated feminist values in their perspectives on work and in their private lives. Work and job are regarded as arising from economic necessity, particularly in inflationary times, and from the breakdown of the family.

Such gender-based issues as traditional roles centered around familial responsibilities, a privatized sense of self, and a restricted view of work may explain why women from traditional families find it particularly difficult to adapt to the role expectations of public sector retraining programs. These job-training programs are heavily oriented towards the male worker, as they address the needs of the labor market. Although the training is task-specific, very little consideration is given to childcare needs or the female client's life situation. Many women have been in nonskilled positions and have not been on a career path that prepared them for job mobility. When they lose their jobs, their work experience is so limited that they are competing with newcomers to the job market. They are, thus, competing with younger persons, their work experience is disregarded, or they are offered entry-level employment and wages.

What is referred to as the "feminization of poverty" (Hartmann, 1987; Lefkovitz & Withorn, 1986; Smith, 1984) can be observed within this population. Demoralization and psychological depression emerge from this situation. The sense of powerlessness observed among women who face the prospects of competing in the job market may stem from their absence of motivational energy to follow a career path. Their self-presentation skills and affect may appear as indifference with regard to exploring vocational direction and options. What these women are in fact communicating is a feeling of inadequacy stemming from their inexperience in seeking work, particularly after several years of secure employment.

There are also women who initiate job change from either the homemaker role or from "high burnout" occupations such as teaching, nursing, and the social services. These women struggle with the stressors associated with a disruption in their career paths. These may include economic insecurity, loss of familiar surroundings, and the struggle with the redefinition of a professional identity. Other women, influenced by the feminist movement, are seeking career opportunities in such fields as finance and management. They often enter these occupations with the desire to abandon the traditional women's work role expectations. These older roles are characterized by an emphasis on nurturance and often require an "unpracticed" presentation of self.

Women under age 35 have been prepared for this transition in professional roles because of their early socialization and education. Job satisfaction, for example, has become more clearly associated with overall life satisfaction for these women because of their explicit career goals. Internal and external obstacles do exist, however, for middle-aged women at mid-career. These women are entering an unfamiliar environment characterized by projected nonfeminine attributes. They perceive the corporate workplace as a less safe and a more competitive environment, albeit one with higher status than the school, the hospital, and the social service agency. The competition for entry into these work environments at mid-career is particularly difficult because young, professionally trained women are choosing legal, financial, and managerial careers upon graduation from college.

The working-class women in both skilled and unskilled occupations, by contrast, frequently do not make the requisite commitment to the occupational role. This is not to say that they do not perform within the job or meet their employers' expectations. They exhibit a sense of pride in their performance, despite their lack of job gratification. From a developmental perspective, having a job had been traditionally viewed by these women as a temporary phase, either prior to marriage or to supplement the family income. Their view of work life as a transitional stage inhibits them from committing to vocational and skill training.

A woman who is ambivalent about working, therefore, faces a crisis when she loses both her job and the security attributed to the longer-term occupational tenure. She must face the reality of her continued need to work. Her skills, however, are less transferable, and her job-seeking abilities are likewise limited. In addition, she may not be confronting the reality that her choice came out of immediate economic necessity rather than longer-range goal orientation. Many such women had left formal education in their adolescence, married or had children at an early age, and were required to work to supplement family income. They held jobs with no career ladder during their working lives; therefore, job transitions present many frustrations for them because of the reality of labor market competition.

Counseling programs for these women need to take into account the differential attitudes towards work roles among professionally and nonprofessionally oriented clientele. Such interventions can reinforce a woman's sense of her value as a worker, and the validity of her contribution to the well-being of the family and to herself, through her work. This is necessary because many working women experience a diminished sense of self as a result of being employed, unlike men who regard work as central to their identities (Hochschild, 1983).

Women's earlier socialization focused on marriage and the family as idealized life goals. However, the power and control over their environment that these women experience in the home are often absent in the workplace. This sense of powerlessness at work results in perceived inadequacy that is exacerbated by job loss. Unlike the men who have been laid off, these women suffer depressive symptoms and, at times, express anger over having to seek employment. There is often an accompanying sense of shame over their lack of skill and the necessity to earn money. The therapist needs to (1) help these women understand the sources of their anger and depression; (2) encourage them to verbalize beliefs regarding their self-concept and attitude toward the work role; and (3) help them become aware of the objective reality that women contribute economically as wage-earners in both two-income families and female-headed households. Although women are certainly aware of the changes that have occurred in family patterns during the course of their lives, they may not have personalized this knowledge.

Counseling interventions can serve to develop the realization of their changed roles. The roles for which they have been socialized have been modified to include a variety of functions.

The changed female role constellation consists of the multiple roles of daughter, wife, mother, and worker. Women are familiar with the problems involved in balancing conflicting and often exhausting role expectations. Through the exploratory process during career transition, these interventions can help female clients acknowledge their inherent strengths and thereby assist them to increase their self-esteem and abilities to cope with transitional stress.

By mid-life, many women have experienced other losses, such as disruption in their marriages, that have required them to function in more autonomous roles. The experience of job loss triggers unresolved conflicts regarding dependency, abandonment, autonomy, and security (Weiss, 1975). Many of these women initially entered full-time employment because of divorce. They frequently accepted menial jobs because they had not worked for some years, or needed jobs that were close to their homes and families. The anger they harbored toward the forced role change as wage-earners is reignited by job loss. At first, they may consciously see the connection between their current feelings of loss and the unresolved conflicts surrounding marital breakup (Wallerstein & Kelly, 1980). By assisting these women to understand their current reactions, they will begin to connect their present and past experiences of loss and change. The loss of their job stirs up their residual anger toward their family or ex-spouse for placing them in a situation where they are responsible for their own support, and often for the decline in their socioeconomic status.

Women clients and, in particular, displaced homemakers, may be discriminated against because of their perceived lack of motivation. They are often viewed as dependent, demanding and thereby "unworthy" of the vocational counselor's efforts. Very often, depressed women clients are viewed as poor candidates for job placement. Vocational counselors often have difficulty understanding that their affect is psychologically rooted. The vocational counselor may build up a defense mechanism of avoidance towards troubled clients that stems from his or her own frustrations in assisting them.

The mental health consultant needs to be alert, therefore, to behavioral signs of depression such as difficulty making decisions, misplaced resentment, pessimism, and low affect among displaced women workers. After such diagnostic efforts, the intervention plan is twofold. The first part is direct service to the troubled client who presents with such depressed symptoms. When a client appears to be clinically depressed, referrals for ongoing care should be made to a community agency. Situational depression can be managed in shorter-term interventions. It is important to point out to the situationally depressed client the possible sources of these reactions. It is also helpful to inform the client of the effect of her demeanor on vocational counselors and other program staff. The concept of "self-fulfilling prophecy" is a useful device for this purpose, because the client will regard herself as unemployable and unworthy of efforts on her behalf. The mental health consultant's second task involves helping the vocational counselor to understand the dynamics of the troubled woman client. The counselors have been trained in assessing the client's vocational skills. Their work experience has taught them to predict which clients are more likely to successfully follow through with the recommendations. They are not always aware of their set responses to psychologically troubled clients.

Mental health consultation should, therefore, focus on the vocational counselor's attitudes towards: (1) the woman client; (2) her self-presentation; (3) her difficulties in communicating her needs; and (4) her barriers toward change. Such consultation should address the counselor's attitudes of frustration and discomfort in breaking through the client's masking, fear of failure, and possible resentment of professionals and bureaucratic personnel. The successful consultation will disclose the unconscious assumptions which bias the vocational counselor's efforts. A change in the vocational counselor's attitudes can bring about a closer, more trusting relationship with the woman client. The successful consultation, therefore, develops better understanding on the part of the client of her own personal reactions to job loss, and on the part of the counselor more skill in helping the client to overcome the emotional obstacles impeding successful outcome in reemployment efforts.

The attributes projected on female clients are essentially negative. These include labels of learned helplessness, shyness and inhibition, motivational deficiency, emotional lability, family-centeredness as opposed to work-centeredness, and other gender-biased perceptions. These attributions are held by women and men in bureaucratic settings. The changes occurring in the economic structure have resulted in shifts in patterns of employment and in job-market expectations. The bias inherent in employment and training programs is on the needs of the male client who is regarded as the principal wage-earner regardless of the economic reality that women represent a major segment of primary wage-earners. Despite the feminist movement, there is an attitudinal lag between past and present economic realities. Mental health professionals in displaced worker programs can influence institutional and individual attitudes toward women, as well as strengthen the coping capacities of the woman client.

EFFECTS OF JOB LOSS ON THE FAMILY

The primary source of stress for the family is economic, that is, the threat to the financial stability of the family. In divorced families, this economic threat extends to child support payments and, therefore, there are ramifications beyond the worker's immediate household. It may also affect available financial support to dependent elderly family members and to offspring who are completing their education. In the single-parent household with a marginal income, there may be a sudden drop in income, since many of these families just manage from paycheck to paycheck. All of these consequences are self-evident; however, their effects evolve over time from the threat of the event, through the various stages of separation, loss, and the resolution of the crisis. The following case illustrates a family's struggle to cope with the crisis of job loss by mobilizing the inherent strengths and competencies of its members without clinical intervention.

CASE: FUNCTIONAL FAMILY COPING

This 50-year-old sound engineer, Harry, lost his job because the company was closing its west coast operation. It was a family decision to remain in California rather then relocate to the east coast, where he was offered a transfer within the same company. Employment opportunities in his field were limited. His age was an obstacle in this highly competitive industry. He was the principal wage-earner in the family. Harry had always been interested in the medical field and made a decision to retrain as a respiratory therapist. He entered a local community college program with the sanction of the immediate family. They readjusted their lifestyle in order to financially support his career change. Harry worked part-time in a hospital and his wife, for the first time in their marriage, took a full-time sales job in a nearby retail shopping mall.

This was a scenario that required the couple to share a sense of high motivation, task-orientation, and psychological competence. It also described a family that had moderate economic resources to sustain itself during the transition, and strong family stability. Of the three children in the family at the point of career transition, the older daughter had completed college and was married; the second child, a son, changed his career goals from acting to retail sales; and a third child, a daughter living in another city, was alienated from the family. The interdependence in this family was between the couple, even though throughout their 25 years of marriage the wife had assumed the stereotypic homemaker role and had, in fact, suffered many attacks of psychosomatic illness very much related to their initial relocation from the east coast. Harry, as the breadwinner, assumed a patriarchal role within this family system. When confronted with the crisis of job loss during middle adulthood, he was furious over his displacement from a "permanent" position. Harry thought through the situation and resisted a transfer, recognizing the disruptive effect it was likely to have on his wife. He examined his options, explored job opportunities, and formulated a strategy that required retraining in a field that was in high demand and that reflected a long-held vocational interest.

Family therapists, such as Minuchin (1974) and Bowen (1971, 1978), would observe that the father in this family was pivotal in maintaining its stability during crisis. In the dysfunctional family, the family therapist might attempt to develop a cohesive alliance between the two adults. To be effective, this alliance would have to accommodate the complementary needs of the couple. In this case, Harry had strong and highly developed nurturant characteristics which served to anchor the family as a unit. His wife regarded herself as fragile, weak, and unable to fulfill the multiple roles of mother, wife, and wage-earner. There were, however, complementary needs being met within this alliance for nurturance and dependency. From the perspective of competence, Harry was able and capable of supporting the family, and weathering the job transition. His wife entered the workplace as a retail clerk and progressed to a supervisory position in what is regarded as an acceptable woman's work role.

Harry and his wife subscribed to a common work ethos, that was socialized within the family, and differentially incorporated by each of the children. The son was strongly identified with his father and, after college and a brief period of experimenting in the film industry, he took a job in the same retail store as his mother and moved up into middle-management. The daughters demonstrated more conflict with respect to the work role. The high-achieving daughter, who was academically successful, married young, had a child, and has, thus far, not entered the world of work. The younger daughter, unable to cope with the conflicting messages in the family, is leading a deviant life. She is a waitress in a small eastern college town and she is alcoholic.

Harry's adaptational process was a synthesis of his strengths, including a pragmatic problem-solving style which had thus far facilitated his establishing and maintaining a stable life structure. This life structure included the necessity to cope with such situations as managing within the constraints of a moderate single-family income, illnesses in the family, substance abuse problems of the youngest child, and the other usual stresses of family life. These adaptational patterns, then, were mobilized during the crisis brought about by job loss.

This family did not receive mental health services at the point at which Harry's career faced the crisis of job loss. Family members routinely coped with stressful events in their lives by using their family physician to treat somatic disorders. Harry's sense of competence, which derived from his own background, helped him to weather this crisis personally. This is an example of a person who was able to mobilize the strengths within him (Katz & Bender, 1976) and, therefore, had no critical need to access mental health services in the community. The following case is an example of a family that had the need to access professional mental health services at the point of crisis, where job loss was the critical event.

CASE: DYSFUNCTIONAL FAMILY COPING

The family consisted of a 42-year-old man who had been divorced and had recently filed for bankruptcy after the failure of a fast-food franchise. After being financially successful for a number of years, the cumulative effects of work-related stress and alcohol use led to the loss of both the marriage and the business. Phil was recovering from this crisis through participation in AA when he met the woman who became his wife. Sandra was in her early thirties with a six-year-old child, and was also divorced and reorganizing her life after a series of life events, including alienation from her family, early substance abuse, and marital breakup. She was successfully employed in a white-collar industry when she met her new husband. After three months of marriage, when layoffs occurred in her company, Sandra lost her job. She was three months pregnant and at a crisis point, because of the convergence of her job loss and her husband's decision to go to school to complete his undergraduate education and make a significant career change. The unplanned but accepted pregnancy exacerbated the crisis of job loss because it affected Sandra's employability, the loss of benefits, and her contribution to the financial support of the family during her husband's career change.

The marital relationship underwent strain as a result of these circumstances, with her husband distancing himself through increased out-of-home activities. This resulted in Sandra's feeling abandoned by Phil, so that job loss became an even more frightening event. The AA program remained a source of common support for this couple and provided some anchorage during this crisis. Their needs as a couple, however, were not adequately met within this self-help group framework. As the pregnancy advanced, Sandra was unable to pursue any job-search activities because of discrimination towards pregnant women who enter the labor market. Phil persisted in his goals by enrolling in the university and refusing to delay his career-change activities despite the pressure of the family's needs.

Sandra sought mental health services in order to counter the threat to her psychological well-being. Her daughter had begun to manifest signs of stress, such as anxious clinging, excessive activity, and sleeplessness. All of this was impacting upon the family's capacity to function. Since this family was a relatively new unit, role definitions had not been fully developed. Each of the adult members had a prior history of psychological dysfunction. They were still in the process of coalescing as a family when the crises, the pregnancy and job loss, took place. They had no past experience in working through such crises as a couple, and prior to this, each had failed to resolve problems because of maladaptive coping styles, such as serious drinking.

Sandra's three-year and Phil's five-year 12-Step-program success experiences had brought them to a more effective, though fragile, place in their lives. Sandra's job loss and pregnancy, as dual crises, were accurately perceived threats to both the marriage and each spouse's individual functioning. Her newly developed self-esteem was strongly linked to her job. This sense of competence in her work carried her through the loss of her job, since she was confident that she could find another job that would use her skills.

The first task of the therapist was diagnostic, and since this was a newly formed family, it was necessary to get a sense of each spouse's idiosyncratic patterns that were brought to the marriage. Phil brought the injuries and failures of both his prior marriage and his economic bankruptcy. He was struggling to move forward in a positive new direction characterized by sobriety, a choice of occupation that involved less risk and lower stress, and his commitment to the new family. Sandra brought a chaotic life history characterized by a dysfunctional family background, including a history of mental illness of a sibling, a recent death of another sibling's defective child, and her own rebellious adolescence which resulted in early marriage, divorce, and substance abuse. Sandra had been working toward stability in her own life through sobriety, a job in a high-status service company, and becoming a responsible adult and parent to her daughter. Together, the couple was working toward a more normalized lifestyle characterized by love, interdependency, and a new start.

The therapist's second task was to help Sandra to be clearer in her observations. Since she was feeling so vulnerable and so needy in her situation, Sandra was reading Phil's self-absorption as rejection. Even though she objectively understood that the loss of her job was part of a general reduction of the company's work force, Sandra was beginning to blame herself for her situation. Phil, on the other hand, was feeling overwhelmed by the financial and emotional demands placed on him. This crisis brought back his feelings of inadequacy and fears of entrapment by the needs of others. His customary style had been to withdraw, use alcohol, and avoid confrontation. In this situation, he refused to be distracted from his career goals. The therapist assisted him in helping Sandra understand and support these longer-term goals as shared goals. They were then able to do some problem-solving regarding immediate financial needs. As a couple, they were strongly motivated to put into practice skills that they had learned in the 12-Step program. The therapist assisted them to reflect on these shared goals, to acknowledge the newness of their relationship, and to recognize that there were many strengths in the marriage. Sandra pursued therapy to help her understand and deal with her own emotional needs during a problem pregnancy. She also began to strengthen her own social support network so that she could decrease her dependency on Phil to meet all of her social and emotional needs. Phil followed through on his educational and career path.

The above case examples show two redirective modes of crisis management. The functional family used a style of crisis resolution that emerged from the problem-solving capabilities and competencies of the family members. The dysfunctional family required the intervention of a therapist to help redirect family members in the face of crisis. According to Rutter (1987), psychosocial resilience to a stressful life event appears to be related to these processes: (1) the reduction of risk impact through cognitive appraisal and alteration of exposure to the risk situation; (2) reduction of negative chain reactions; (3) self-esteem and self-efficacy through personal relationships and task accomplishments; and (4) opportunities and turning points in people's lives when a risk trajectory may be redirected onto a more adaptive path. In the more functional family, the risks that accompany job loss as a stressful life event are mediated by mobilizing familial and community-support systems, intrafamilial communication and decision-making strengths, and redirection of the family member at risk into a positive action framework.

LIFE COURSE AND WORK IDENTITY

Job loss occurs for each person at a different point in life and its effect appears to be closely related to when it occurs in a person's life. Levinson's model of adult development divides the life course into eras and developmental periods and relates these stages to crisis and change (Levinson, 1979, 1986). We will assess the impact of job loss as a life crisis during each stage of the adult life cycle, using Levinson's model, as a family crisis, and as an individual event.

During the transition to early adulthood (17 to 22), the process of emancipation from the family of origin and preparation for an occupational path are central tasks. Job loss during this transition has limited, if any, impact on the individual. However, as the individual enters the world of young adulthood (22 to 28), frequently accompanied by marriage and the beginning of a new family unit, job loss may be a disruptive event to a person's sense of competence and to the family's economic and psychosocial stability. For the young adult who may be living on her or his own for the first time, this event may threaten this newly found autonomy. In many situations, this young adult must return, because of economic necessity, to the family of origin. This may disrupt the household to which she or he returns, as there are pressures involved in restructuring family relationships to accommodate the change. Job loss creates an imbalance and tests the capability to cope with crisis for the young couple in this stage who are in the process of developing an interdependent relationship. Decisions, such as family planning, geographical relocation, training, and education, force these individuals to assume adult responsibilities. Many may have been unprepared to anticipate job loss at this stage and are, therefore, both emotionally and economically unprepared for this contingency within the family.

Blue-collar workers between ages 22 and 28 facing layoff have begun working directly out of high school for larger companies in unskilled and semiskilled occupations. They developed their work skills on the job and in many instances managed to progress within the company. These younger workers derived a sense of security that comes from working in a setting in which they were accepted and were able to progress in a place that was virtually noncompetitive. After layoff, these individuals enter a more competitive job market requiring a better educational background. For the more introspective youth, self-examination regarding opportunities for post-secondary education and skill development are paramount during this stage, and these individuals will often move on to another company after layoff.

This dichotomy—between structured and serendipitous perceptions of career goals— brings about two very different styles of relating to job loss. Job loss for the mindful individual represents a disruption in a newly arrived-at structure. This may have been a person's first, or perhaps second, job and that person may have been in a workplace for between four and seven years, and may have been anchored by the work. This is a particularly disrupting event if that person has been completing an emancipation process from the family of origin by forming a new family and thereby establishing an independent adult identity. For the serendipitous person, by contrast, job loss engenders a sense of withholding and denial which comes about from an internal lack of clarity regarding career goals. This style may be characteristic of many individuals who, at this stage, have yet to focus seriously on longer-term occupational goals. The following case illustrates how job loss can revive longer-standing personal conflicts that may severely limit a person's sense of competence and thereby deter the successful resolution of the crisis, namely, reemployment.

CASE

Jennifer was a 24-year-old unmarried woman who lost her job in a large retail sales outlet after working there for four years. This event revived conflicts around her achievement and the problems she had encountered with her education. She expressed feelings of confusion, she was depressed, and she was suffering from anxiety because of low self-esteem and self-doubt about entering a training program. She had experienced personal conflict throughout the four years of her employment over what she regarded as being a low-status occupation. She had been encouraged by her family to pursue a college education and she had attempted to do this by registering for courses at a local community college but then dropping out before completing them. Health problems interfered with her capacity to balance work and schooling. The erratic work hours imposed by the retail sales position made it difficult also for her to plan part-time attendance at school. Jennifer blamed herself for what she perceived as a series of personal failures, including her lack of persistence in fulfilling academic goals. She was currently offered an opportunity, through a federal job training program, to develop new skills, but she was apprehensive once again about failure. She recognized her need for mental health counseling during this crisis, although she viewed her prior treatment experiences as not being helpful.

Jennifer sought career/vocational assessment to help clarify her goals. Educational and cognitive assessment was also recommended. She was encouraged to seek therapy and a referral was made to a community setting where both her emotional and vocational problems would be addressed. Jennifer was a young person who had been attempting to create a stable life structure economically in order to emancipate herself from her family of origin. She had not, however, resolved personal conflicts regrading school failure and, as a bright middle-class young woman, had not addressed the disparities between her personal values and goal expectations, and the reality of her work life. The symptom formation of psychosomatic disorders, emotional lability, and recurrent depression surfaced at this crisis point in her life.

The Age-30 Transition and the ensuing Settling-Down Period (33 to 40) bring about an expansion in the focus of family concerns and responsibilities to include a trigenerational perspective. These concerns include perceiving oneself as an adult, the multiple tasks of parenting, concerns of becoming parents, and enhanced involvement and identification with the parental generation. In this society, the awareness of being an adult comes into sharper focus for those at the age-30 transition, at which point the individual is expected to be well along the path to a stable career direction. Job loss, at this time, does not usually involve much of a shift in vocational direction. A person who expected to remain working in a company where advancement possibilities were good and a career ladder existed is likely to be thrown off balance by job loss. There are many individuals, however, who chose particular career tracks which were not gratifying and who, during a crisis at this age, begin to examine their options. Those who are less committed to a specific occupation or work setting have less difficulty in accepting job loss and experience less personal loss. Those individuals who dropped out of school and went into lower-skilled jobs and serendipitously moved along an occupational track frequently experience frustration regarding available options.

Women who had been socialized to believe that work outside the home would be only a temporary activity, rather than a significant part of their adult life, are forced into confronting a different reality. Many were not prepared for work and a career because of socialized attitudes of their families toward women's work role as solely an economic necessity. For women whose interests are more "home-centered," job loss poses a dilemma of either refocusing their activities back into the home setting, which may be their wish, or acknowledging the necessity of their employment. These women will often experience conflicting feelings of anger and depression over the loss of their income, ambivalent feelings over a change in status from full-time worker to homemaker, and a sense of relief from not having to work outside the home. For women who are more ego-involved in their careers and have clear vocational goals, the transition to a new job is often seen as a challenge and an opportunity for personal and career growth. Conflicts within the family system will often parallel the displaced worker's emotional reactions to the crisis of job loss, as in the following case example of a man at this stage who experiences life changes.

CASE

Barry is a man in his early thirties who lost his job because of the corporate takeover of a large retail sales chain where he was employed. Although he was underemployed in terms of his career aspirations, this job with its flexible work hours had allowed him to attend the local university where he was nearing the completion of a degree in computer science. Barry was extremely angry about job loss occurring at this point in his life. His personal life had become unstable due to a recent divorce and his responsibility for the support of one child.

Job loss and the breakup of the marriage triggered strong emotional reactions. Barry's early education had been interrupted as a result of his family's immigration to the United States from Western Europe. His personal sense of helplessness was intensified by these multiple loss experiences. As a highly motivated person, he had been able to combine work and school with his family life. He was disillusioned and bitter about the disintegration of his life structure, and he found himself immobilized and thereby powerless to plan for his immediate future. He was reluctant to seek a new job that would interfere with the completion of his education, even though it was an economic necessity. His behavior was belligerent when he was offered either job placement or training opportunities in a lower-level job. His conflict was whether to commit to a career path that would use the skills he was developing at the university, or to find a job similar to the one he had lost, which would make few demands upon him and thereby allow him to compete his final coursework at the university.

Barry was resistant to counseling during this crisis. The recommendations offered to him were rejected because of his distrust of authority, resulting from disillusionment and pain. He needed to regain his sense of personal empowerment that was threatened by the recent circumstances over which he had no control. His anger and depression seemed linked to his obsessive-compulsive character structure which made change in general difficult to accept. Greater personal flexibility would have helped him to adapt to this interruption of his current life agenda. The lack of a stable support system placed him at risk. Although in need of psychological counseling, Barry rigidly resisted any perceived intrusion into his personal life situation. Barry was in the midst of the age-30 transition. This period is conceptualized as a time for reflection and examination of past opportunities and prior decisions regarding educational, vocational, and career choices. Barry's personal life situation was too chaotic for him to feel comfortably reflective. He chose to seek employment in a non-challenging job and pursue the completion of his academic goals.

Job loss and reemployment during the settling-down stage (ages 33 to 40) are often characterized by the principal wage-earner making a relatively rapid transition from one job to another. This is a change point that tests an individual's and a family's adaptive style. The behavioral consequences of individual career change in the family setting may include an increased level of irritability, distractibility, and perhaps preoccupation with workplace issues. There is an interruption in an individual's everyday life routine that results from concerns about succeeding in the new job. The need for increased levels of emotional support and understanding from other family members is often overlooked during this transition. These increased needs, however, can be accommodated in the more functional family. Any change in a highly stressed family disrupts the balance within that system. Adapting to this transition of the principal wage-earner who is most often regarded as having the power to maintain the family's stability requires family members to acknowledge and address that person's emotional demands.

In a dual-career family, the crisis brought about by job change may be economically less disruptive than in the single wage-earner family. Each member of the dyad shares a familiarity with workplace issues, including risks, transitions, and adjustment processes. These perceptions of the work role in a period of major structural economic change are thus jointly recognized and experienced. In the single wage-earner family, by contrast, unless there has been open communication regarding workplace issues and family roles, the displaced worker may experience a sense of isolation and, in some instances, that her or his role in the family has been undermined. A similar threat in the dual-career family is the setback in the pattern of success, which may lead to criticism and judgmental attribution by the spouse with the stable job. Resentments may build because the economic life of the family, which was shared, is less equitable to the sole wage-earner. This appears to be a greater problem when it is the husband who has lost his job, because of traditional role expectations.

Turning 40 in the United States in the late 1980s has received a great deal of attention because of multiple factors, including media influences, marketing strategies, and current psychological trends toward life-span developmental theories (Nichols, 1986). The age-40 transition, in Levinson's developmental paradigm, describes the individual's moving toward fulfillment of earlier goals and ambitions. Typical life crises center around the marriage, choice of career, and questioning of sources of gratification and personal values. The need at this transition stage for a personal sense of empowerment is closely tied to achievement. An individual's socioeconomic reality—as defined by lifestyle, career, and success measured by financial rewards and other status indicators—has a greater impact during this transition now that emancipation or autonomy needs are no longer in the forefront.

In major corporations, individuals in this age cohort are overly represented in middle-management, and the more successful tend to strongly identify with the workplace and its values. For skilled and semiskilled workers, including those employed in service industries, work and the job have different attributes. Employees in their early forties are struggling with changing work conditions, including shrinking advancement opportunities, less job security, increasing specialization, and the diminished power of labor unions. These unsettling conditions in turn affect interpersonal relationships and mirror the turbulence in the contemporary family. For the individual this may become a period of mid-life crisis. A successful resolution of this crisis depends upon a person's sense of job gratification, support system strength, and family integration. Job loss at this life transition can be an extreme stressor. When the life event comes about precipitously, the individual's sense of power and control is challenged.

CASE

Dan was a displaced auto worker in his early forties. He was married with two children and lived in the same working-class suburban community in which he grew up. He had been employed as an assembly worker for 17 years. His marriage had withstood the many years of Dan's alcoholism preceding his entering a 12-Step program. His early school failure was attributed to dyslexia, which was diagnosed concurrent with his son's learning disability.

His wife took a job outside the home when the children were in their early adolescence. In addition to his assembly work, Dan had become one of the plant's peer substance abuse counselors, and this provided him with a sense of pride in achievement. Because of his multiple early problems, Dan's employment options were limited. Despite these setbacks, his motivation to succeed was not destroyed. When the plant closed and he was laid off, he began to receive unemployment insurance and supplemental union benefits. He continued to work "on the side" in auto repair, as he had always done to supplement his income. Because of his peer counseling experience, he was offered a temporary position with the union. When the company formally announced the permanent plant closure, Dan was faced with the choice of relocating out of state or relinquishing accrued retirement benefits, with over 17 years vested in his pension plan.

This became the crisis in Dan's life that he was forced to resolve at age 43. He had strong roots in his community, responsibility for his mother and mother-in-law, and concern for his son's special educational needs and his wife's medical problems. This crisis was unlike previous transitions in his life during which Dan avoided dealing with conflict and resorted to excessive acting-out behaviors when under stress. With the sense of responsibility and maturity achieved at age 43, and fortified by the knowledge that he had acquired experientially through Alcoholics Anonymous (AA), Dan was able to examine his options and struggle through a difficult decision-making process.

Dan's family was supportive, although they clearly stated that they preferred not to relocate. At one point, he decided that he would relocate to a midwestern city, live alone, and visit his family in California for long weekends and holidays for the next seven years, after which he would be eligible for retirement. This plan thrust him and the family into a crisis. Fortunately, a job offer came along through his AA network that resulted in a challenging new position. The crisis, occurring at this age, was difficult because of the complexities of his family life, personal attachments, and responsibilities. The life experiences and skills which led to his personal integration at age 43, however, enabled him to make a successful transition.

THE DISPLACED OLDER WORKER

Losing one's job during the era of middle adulthood (45 to 60) has a varying impact on an individual's well-being. The impact appears to be dependent upon such factors as financial stability, career path, transferability of skills, and the perception that one's internal and external environments are coherent (Antonovsky, 1979, 1987). By this time an individual has usually achieved a stable work life, which includes a mastery of skills, promotion to supervisory or managerial responsibility, and job stability. Women who have entered the labor market after the childbearing years have usually found a career role by this age. There are, however, many individuals who do not achieve this stable point in the lives for a variety of economic, social, and psychological reasons.

Individuals who have achieved tenure or seniority, through either civil service or union protection, are unprepared when job loss occurs. When these so-called "secure jobs" are lost, these workers' overall sense of stability is shattered, often resulting in significant stress reactions. Early retirement is rarely an option for those in this stage of life for both economic and personal reasons. The more skilled worker and the professional have greater options during the transition. Being out of work, looking for a job and marketing one's skills at this life stage of life present both a challenge and a threat.

Many older workers have expressed the positive view that they had been considering a change anyway because they were "in a rut." Others have stated that the security offered by their jobs had prevented them from initiating change. Some were bitter and blamed themselves for not having made a change earlier in their lives. For those who had found their niche, job loss was a disruptive force in their lives.

CASE

Bill was a married man in his late forties who had been employed by a retail merchandising chain for 15 years. He was assistant manager and supervisor at the time of the layoff. This unionized company provided a good wage and benefit package to its employees. It had become a successful chain of retail stores when it was acquired in a corporate takeover, resulting in mass layoffs. Bill was not introspective; his style of communicating his feelings was nondisclosing and restricted to superficial details. He was among the first group to be terminated from the company, although all of the company's employees would eventually lose their jobs. This event was traumatic for Bill and his self-esteem. Job loss resulted in a sense of personal powerlessness. This impeded Bill's capacity to initiate activities that would lead to finding work.

Bill had progressed within the company to a supervisory position. He had a sense of achievement in what he perceived as a secure position with good benefits. The loss of the job at this point in his life brought about a loss of balance. Bill was thrust into a competitive labor market without the feeling of competence and emotional armor present in the younger men whom he saw as his competition. He was well adapted to his job loss and expressed an intense sense of despair and disappointment over the closing of this store. His self-image was closely identified with his former workplace and his role as a manager, and it was very difficult for him to conceive of another job for which he would be hired at his previous level. Bill needed to financially support himself and his wife, but he was having difficulty mobilizing for a serious job search. The training programs offered to Bill neither interested him nor seemed to be practical options. They were unappealing because they were in computer-related fields and his work skills were primarily service-and management-oriented.

Bill had become depressed and anxious, experienced sleep disturbances, and was feeling immobilized. He enrolled in a federally funded reemployment program that included career dynamics and job-search workshops, and interaction with other displaced workers. These activities helped decrease his social isolation. During a group session, Bill disclosed his feelings of shame at being without a job. He claimed to have avoided both the company of former co-workers as well as public places in his community where he would be likely to meet former customers. Bill's sense of personal identity was threatened in a manner that can be compared to that of the "displaced homemaker" who, prior to divorce or widowhood, regarded herself as economically secure in the role of a wife, and then was thrust unwillingly into making a life change.

The goal of intervention with members of this age group is to explore the available options in the current labor market that utilize the cumulative work experiences of clients with a history of job stability. Bill's active participation in the support groups helped him to rebuild his sense of self-esteem and purpose. These strengths enabled him to maximize the use of a supportive network of family, friends, and peers to help find new employment. Once Bill was able to present himself in his former sociable and affable manner, he could then reestablish those ties necessary in any job search.

In a society that values youth, a person of this age encountering change experiences fear of rejection and diminished worth (Butler, 1975). The perception that one's personal attributes are devalued is apparent even in a middle-aged person who is highly skilled, perhaps professionally trained, and with recognized competence. The traumatic effects of job loss are devastating because of the multiple role obligations and expectations of persons in this age group. The indicators of transitional stress prevalent in this group are anxiety, depression, and sleep disturbances. The increased use of alcohol is particularly evident, as former co-workers will often maintain their former social ties through drinking together.

Family relationships, particularly spousal bonds, are threatened by job loss at this stage. How the couple pulls together through this crisis depends on the strength of the bond, trust, and perceived self-efficacy (Bandura, 1977, 1982). Successful transition rests on the ability of the individual to mobilize and successfully pursue, follow through, and be future-oriented. The attitude of the spouse appears to be central to self-confidence, morale, and successful adaptation. A man's sense of self-efficacy is often linked to his spouse's expression of confidence that he will find new employment. A woman's sense of self-esteem is less linked to her career, as is that of a man of this age. There are many women, in fact, who welcome job loss at this stage of life, viewing it as an opportunity to shift careers or to become more home-based. The economic issues, however, for the primary wage-earner and head of household are the same for both men and women.

The age-50 transition (ages 50 to 55), within this life stage, when complicated by job loss, throws the person's life into disequilibrium. The structure-changing periods in Levinson's model are times when the person has the opportunity to modify and to improve the "entry life structure" of a particular era, in this case, middle adulthood. The forced change brought about by job loss interferes, in this conceptual model, with the individual's sense of stability. A person requires the stability of a secure job in order to reflect upon current achievement and place in the world. This "safe base" securely anchors a person to a point from which she or he can consider where she or he is in life, work, and career. The precipitous loss of job puts this process of change out of balance.

Though many people consider making a change at this point in life, few people voluntarily act on this wish. Obstacles that inhibit conscious risk taking include their fear of change, the presumed security that their jobs provide, and the opportunities they see as being available to them. Risking job change at this age is commonly regarded as hazardous. The sense of being emotionally and economically trapped and the ensuing frustration result in marital discord and emotional upheaval. At this life stage, one usually reflects upon youthful dreams and expectations, including economic goals, occupational achievement, and personal recognition. Losing a job, without the immediate possibility of transition into a position of comparable or higher status, is a threat to a person's sense of self-worth.

Coping effectively with this change taps the individual's strengths that have been developed through life. A person's sense of self-confidence, for example, in the ability to master the age-50 transition is linked to the competence, skills, and sense of empowerment derived from successfully mastering previous life crises. Change, for some people, constitutes a major threat to their well-being. Others perceive it as a challenge and mobilize accordingly. The following cases illustrate two styles of adapting to job loss and career change at the age-50 transition.

CASE

Helen, at age 53, lost her job as a customer service representative at a local retail chain store. She had been working at this job for three years, following early retirement from a municipal civil service job. Her work abilities were varied and included highly developed office skills. Helen had been working since her early adolescence, was self-supporting, and unmarried. This unexpected job loss was a threat to her economic security since her retirement income was insufficient to maintain her lifestyle, including the support of an aging parent. Despite these factors, she had good morale and high self-esteem and confidence in her capacity to secure a good job. She was considering participating in a training program that would provide her with updated skills using computerized automated office machines. Helen had planned to remain at her job until her retirement, thus assuring income from two pension plans; however, personal resilience, optimism, and sense of competence were strengths that she tapped to adjust to this transition and to modify her life structure.

Grace was a 53-year-old executive secretary to an industrial plant manager. She was discharged from her job that she held for nine years when the plant closed. This was the second time that she was affected by plant closure since she had previously worked for 12 years for a mail order distribution firm which went out of business. Grace enjoyed her role as assistant to the company executive and functioned in that role in what has been described as a "corporate wife" (Kanter, 1977). This caretaking role, characterized by deference to and maintenance of the corporate executive's needs, created in Grace a sense of reflected importance. She was well-dressed and attractive, and presented herself as a cut above the other women in the organization. Grace had been recently widowed, and this additional threat to her security and status placed her at high risk for stress reactions. This combination of recent loss of spouse and job displacement, with the accompanying role losses, created a heightened vulnerability. Her prior jobs had required good secretarial and office management skills; however, the personal secretary role has less transferability for a woman of her age in the current job market. Grace's strengths and her unique value to the executive in this company were idiosyncratic; women who are in these corporate situations for a number of years are at a great disadvantage when they seek new employment.

This woman's identity and sense of competence, so strongly attached to being the person upon whom the corporate executive depended, were destroyed when the job ended. She was unable, initially, to consider her options, although she would need to seek other employment or modify her lifestyle considerably. Despite the fact that Grace had many years of work experience, her repertoire of skills was limited and outdated. Grace was a conventional person whose functional adaptation to the "wife role," both at home and at work, was a source of gratification. Her feelings of superiority, derived from the status of her "boss," served to isolate Grace from most of the other women with whom she worked. With the impending job loss, she did not have the social support of her co-workers.

Grace's personal style and rigidity, which were assets in her role as an executive secretary, proved disadvantageous in her job search. Her lack of flexibility was a cause of stress and anxiety in confronting the future. She intended to defer seeking assistance in attaining new employment, choosing rather to spend some time with her married children.

In comparing the cases of Helen and Grace, the significant predictors of successful career transition seem to be flexibility, adaptability, perception of social role with respect to work, and autonomy. These four factors would appear to reflect an individual's sense of competence. The age-50 transition was far more difficult for Grace, whose values and self-image, remained rooted in an earlier generation's definition of the woman's work role. Helen, by comparison, was able to adapt to the less stereotyped image of the working woman. She took risks and valued change, regarding it as a challenge. Helen was less home-centered and, although traditional in her attachments to her family, she was task-oriented in her work, rather than developing strong personal ties to her superiors. Her sources of gratification were through achievement and economic independence.

Men and women in their early fifties face both a challenge and a crisis when job loss threatens their life structure economically and psychologically. The crisis that they can expect to confront—the threat to their self-image, the fear of failure, and the need to compete with younger workers—may bring about stress reactions. Clinicians can best assist these individuals by focusing on their inherent strengths and the coping strategies that have helped them weather previous crises (Rosow, 1974). In this manner, the individual's sense of competence and self-empowerment are reinforced.

THE DISPLACED WORKER FROM A MINORITY ETHNIC SUBCULTURAL GROUP

In recent years, companies have had to demonstrate compliance with federally mandated affirmative action and fair employment regulations. This has entailed active recruitment of both American-born ethnic subcultural group members and newly arrived refugees from Southeast Asia and Central America. A large number of workers from ethnic subcultural groups entered the workplace at the time that these regulations were being actively enforced. The expansion of such industries as electronic assembly offered many newly arrived immigrants from Southeast Asia and Central America employment opportunities. It was often unnecessary for these monolingual individuals to develop or improve their English language skills or to develop transferable job skills. During this expansionary period, monolingual Asian and Latino workers had opportunities to move laterally from one electronic company to another, and they frequently lived among other newly arrived immigrants in refugee communities. These two factors, coupled with long working hours, shift work conditions, and home and family responsibilities, inhibited their opportunities for upward job mobility which is dependent upon work skill and English-language capability.

It has been recognized that many of those from recently arrived immigrant groups—most notably from Asia—have made impressive economic gains. The vulnerable populations, however—lesser-skilled workers—are stratified by their achievement. The Korean woman who has worked for 15 years cleaning fish in a tuna packing house on the Long Beach waterfront may have children who are moving up the economic ladder. But she may be virtually unable to find another job when the packing plant shuts down. The Latino cannery worker, with a 15-year work history, will also find himself unemployable because of limited language skills and nontransferable work skills. By comparison, the few Anglo employees in this plant will have less difficulty in finding a job since the opportunities are greater for them.

The clinician, in working with clients from minority ethnic subcultural groups, must take into account interethnic variation specific to job loss in the following areas: (1) denial systems, pride, and shame arising from job loss; (2) optimism regarding the future; (3) motivation for economic achievement; (4) modes of disclosure, in general, and, specifically, talking about money; (5) familial and social support systems; (6) coping styles; (7) help-seeking strategies; and (8) service utilization (Harwood, 1981).

CASE

Millie had worked for a major urban medical center as a nursing assistant for 12 years until the hospital eliminated her job category. She was 42 years old, the single head of household, living in an inner city Black neighborhood. She had three adult children, two of whom were sons who were recent college graduates. The third was a daughter who had serious emotional and substance abuse problems. Millie was referred to the reemployment center that was sponsored by the local community college. She was receiving unemployment insurance benefits and retained her company's health benefit package. The center offered her educational and vocational assessment, basic skills training, the opportunity to participate in career transition workshops, and a special women's group.

Millie availed herself of all opportunities. She made a commitment toward improving herself and learning new skills. She had worked hard all her life in unskilled jobs to support her family, and she motivated them educationally. Millie was very proud of her sons' achievements, but she was struggling to separate herself from her daughter's addictive behavior, although she helped care for her daughter's child. She was determined to succeed, even at midlife, in a new career. Millie spent four months preparing for her high-school equivalency exam, which she passed, and she entered an automated office machine skills retraining program.

Millie was a reserved and friendly person with a clear sense of direction at this age. She expressed her feelings of having always sacrificed for her family, but of now being able to pursue educational goals that were previously unattainable. She was encouraged by the members of the women's group to strengthen her support system so that she could continue to detach from the mutually destructive relationship with her daughter. Losing her job at the hospital had disrupted her life, but she acknowledged that she would not have initiated a job change due to her feelings of inadequacy. She described the drudgery of her work for those many years and wondered aloud how the hospital was going to maintain adequate patient care without nursing assistants.

Millie's pride of achievement as a mother and as the sole source of economic support of her family gave her the strength to change her work life. She had insight into her educational deficits that needed to be remedied. There were two other women from her former workplace in Millie's group who provided emotional support and encouragement to each other. These supportive ties enabled all three women to sustain the frustration of the initial stages of the reemployment program.

In sum, although ethnic subcultural group differences may impinge upon the clinical reality, understanding clients' competency and attributes may have much relevance in helping them.

JOB LOSS AS A COMMUNITY CRISIS

Policymakers have demonstrated concern about the ever-increasing burden of social welfare programs for the chronically mentally ill and the chronically unemployed. The cost of such programs, such as Aid to Families with Dependent Children (AFDC) and the resentment of taxpayers toward their support have required that policymakers develop alternatives. The involvement of the private sector in these programs indicates its acknowledgment of major structural economic change and an increasing concern for the population of workers at high risk of becoming part of the welfare system. Thus far, programs for the unemployed, specifically displaced workers, have had limited visibility.

Despite the fact that approximately $300 million has been allocated each year since the early 1980s for training and reemploying the recently and longer-term unemployed in California, alone, the plight of displaced workers and their need for psychological services have only been minimally remedied through federally funded programs. By comparison, the federal Disaster Relief Act of 1974, Section 413, acknowledges the need for mental health counseling services when the President declares a state of emergency. Funds then become available to the affected community to provide crisis-counseling services to the disaster victims. This enabling legislation is unique because of its recognition of the effects of sudden psychological trauma on a community. Funds are also available when job loss is caused by a disaster. Ironically, there are no comparable funds made available for the psychological needs of displaced workers. Local mental health authorities have been forced by financial stringencies and limited definitions of eligibility to concentrate their services on the chronically and seriously mentally ill in their communities. Mentally ill homeless individuals thereby become eligible for public mental health programs, and this group is also eligible for federal job-training programs. Preventive mental health programs for displaced workers are limited and are provided only in those communities where there are activists advocating for these services.

Layoffs and plant closures in the major industrial states have to date been relatively isolated events with minimal ripple effects on the macrostructure. The potential for downward socioeconomic mobility is greatest for those workers displaced from sectors of the economy affected by technological change, with unskilled and semiskilled workers being at the highest risk. Many skilled workers are also at risk, since their jobs have been affected by foreign competition and relocation of many industries to the periphery—that is, to those third-world countries undergoing industrialization—because of lower wages and anticipated higher productivity.

An increased number of formerly employed individuals and their families have recently fallen onto hard times as a result of job loss. Similar to the new urban homeless populations in their (a) marginality, (b) lack of job permanence, and (c) lower functional skill levels, these are frequently lower-skilled workers and low wage-earners who are poorly equipped to compete in the new job market. The impact on these individuals who are being confronted with the need to seek assistance from entitlement and unemployment programs, and who foresee the possibility of becoming part of the public welfare system, is often demoralizing. The customary clients of public entitlement programs such as AFDC families, who are headed by women of childbearing age, enter the system at an earlier age and frequently remain there as a result of physical disabilities. The most vulnerable of the displaced workers, by contrast, are entering their middle years, have established an independent lifestyle, and hold a value system that is incongruent with "welfare thinking." Many of these families have been dependent on two wage-earners and have encumbered their projected earnings with car payments and recently acquired homes with high mortgage rates. The ripple effect on the household economy of a person's job loss—either that of the primary wage-earner or a partner in a dual wage-earning family—seriously disrupts the family system.

COMMUNITY SUPPORT: MACROSOCIAL APPROACHES

At the federal level, the legislative concern for displaced workers has led to the creation of federally funded job training programs. Government-subsidized work programs, such as the Works Progress Administration projects, have been in place since the 1930s. These efforts, however, have always been criticized as being ineffective in developing permanent job skills and motivating achievement. In the past, there have been such programs as the Comprehensive Employment Training Act (CETA), which provided stipends and subsidized training and/or employment, often in public sector jobs. Nonprofit community-based organizations (CBO), such as the Urban League and the United Auto Workers, that initially received CETA funds for the training of their own constituencies, expanded their mission to include skill training for involvement in a broader labor market. The Job Training Partnership Act (JTPA) programs, by contrast, involve partnerships between the public and private sectors, attempt to maintain rigidly defined performance standards with respect to placement in new employment, and are without the economic support in the form of stipends to the client.

The JTPA programs of the 1980s involve linkages on the local level among private industry, labor organizations, educational institutions, and local government agencies. The interpretation of government regulations and standards for performance occur at the local level. Training programs are approved and funded on the basis of local labor market analyses. The elaborate administrative structure that underlies JTPA programs emphasizes local control for purposes of planning and spending. The development of policy for the JTPA-funded programs through local private industry councils (PICs) reflects the interests and ideological commitments of the community power structure. Although policy determinations are made at this local level with the intent of fostering a process of decentralized decision-making, the actual control is vested in the city, state, and federal government agencies that are charged with program planning and evaluation of the performance standards of contractors that implement these objectives.

The emergence of local community support on behalf of displaced workers has been minimal, particularly in the Los Angeles metropolitan area, because of the fragmentation and diversity of interests among the local communities within the region. The heterogeneity of the industries that have been affected by plant closures and layoffs and of their work forces has precluded the development of shared interests and community concern for displaced worker issues. When the Bethlehem Steel Corporation closed its Los Angeles plant after a series of layoffs, there were attempts by union members to develop a broader-based coalition of support for displaced workers. They were able to organize a food distribution program collaboratively with other unions in their local region. They were unsuccessful, however, in their efforts at coalition-building. The obstacles to community support in this case were due to the lack of concentration of workers in any one community, the gradual erosion of the work force at the steel mill over a three-to-five-year period, the multiethnic composition of the workers, and the union members' disillusionment with the labor organization as a viable force working on behalf of the interests of displaced workers.

A similar set of circumstances characterized the closing of the General Motors assembly plant in the neighboring industrial community of Southgate. The coalition-building that took place prior to the formal closure of the automobile assembly plant became focused on the economic redevelopment of the urban infrastructure, from an industrial base to an economy based on warehouse and tourism services. The auto workers' identification with the local community was minimal, nor did they identify with the municipality's redevelopment efforts. Their primary relationship was with the plant where they were employed and not with the community itself, despite the fact that the local union hall was located there. Efforts to organize social activities and political rallies were unsuccessful because of the geographic dispersal of the work force. The retired workers, by contrast, tended to reside closer to the plant and, therefore, maintained a stronger affiliation with the union hall as a social center. Organizational efforts on their behalf were impeded by the workers' disillusionment with the local union leadership, their resistance to returning to a union hall across from the deserted factory to which they had commuted from surrounding cities, and their own unformulated identities as displaced workers. The latter condition may be attributed to the fact that the workers were still subject to recall by General Motors, were receiving union-based financial supplements to their unemployment benefits, and therefore held a tenuous status.

The socioeconomic base of the communities in which both the steel mill and automobile assembly plant were located was primarily industrial and composed of low-income, minority residents. These communities had undergone population shifts in recent years from predominantly middle-class industrial workers and their families to households composed of newly arrived monolingual Hispanic immigrants. There was minimal local expression of concern for displaced workers and no local-level initiatives on their behalf. The ripple effect of these plant closures on local small businesses, ranging from restaurants, bars and retail outlets to smaller technical operations such as tool and die works and machine shops that maintained a symbiotic relationship to the large industrial plants, created an economic hardship that was evident in the communities. The displaced workers themselves were perceived by residents as outsiders to the community and as "advantaged" because of the economic safety net provided by their unions. The psychological isolation engendered by these circumstances discouraged alliance-building within the two industrial communities. These commuting workers were alienated from their residential communities as well, since being laid off was an experience that was not shared by their neighbors and friends outside the workplace. This situation reinforced the individualism, as well as, perhaps, a sense of shame and self-blame, that is characteristic of attitudes projected by the public agencies that provide benefits and support to the unemployed.

A plant closure and the resulting worker dislocation occurs as an isolated event, except in single-industry company towns where the event is universally experienced as a community crisis similar to a natural disaster. The impact on the individual in a disaster is shared by other community members and is not a source of stigma. After the disaster event, resources become mobilized, mutual assistance emerges, cohesiveness develops around rescue operations, and sharing of concerns for the severely affected evolves; and all of these efforts strengthen community bonds. Psychological stressors affecting the individual, caused by property loss and residential dislocation, physical injury, and perhaps loss of loved ones, may result in immediate and post-traumatic stress reactions. These reactions, however, are buffered by the presence of a common, nonstigmatized, naturally occurring event such as a disaster.

There are similarities between disaster victims and displaced workers in their psychological responses to the traumatic event. The sense of self-blame that both groups report is related to their perceived loss of control and self-empowerment. The experience of loss of a home, and its resultant physical displacement, has its parallel in the longer-term employee's experience of displacement from the familiar terrain of the workplace. Feelings of sadness and disorientation are reported in both instances. The legitimacy of the disaster victim's perceptions and feelings is reinforced by community institutions; the displaced worker's feelings of loss, by contrast, lack such socially sanctioned legitimacy. It is commonly accepted that separation of the disaster victim from the community is sometimes necessary for the reconstruction of the physical infrastructure. The displaced worker's permanent separation from familiar work surroundings and a "work family" has a similar traumatic effect without the extended community support of common acceptance of these emotional responses to job loss.

COPING STYLES AND ADAPTATION TO JOB LOSS

Technological change has rendered certain forms of work obsolete and has limited employment opportunities in certain key occupations. Aerospace engineers in Southern California during the 1970s, for example, were forced into unemployment. These professionals had been in high demand in the previous two decades and they commanded high salaries. The restructuring of health care in the 1980s displaced licensed vocational

nurses and other hospital workers who had previously experienced labor market demand for their services. Companies
in the film industry, that formerly employed craftspeople like
cartoonists and animators, have relocated this work to the Far
East, thereby eliminating employment opportunities for these
specialized occupational groups. Employees in the garment industry with their specialized skills have also been displaced
by their companies' decisions to manufacture abroad.

The individuals displaced from the aforementioned representative Southern California industries possess highly developed skills and a strong attachment to their work. The
permanent loss of opportunities to work in their chosen fields
has shattered their economic security. The realization of the
loss of their source of livelihood, coupled with the loss of personal fulfillment and meaning derived from the work itself,
has further eroded their well-being. The resulting demoralization of these workers, who must confront these socioeconomic
and personal realities, can both destroy their self-esteem and
impair their sense of future orientation. Their problem-solving
skills that are necessary to resolve this crisis are inhibited as
well by the insult to their image of themselves as competent
and self-sufficient adults.

Despite these circumstances and the different styles of coping with job loss, an individual's capacity to adapt to change
depends upon flexibility, personal competence, and action.
During the course of their working lives, many people change
jobs, return to the workplace after raising a family, or change
careers because of expanded job opportunities. There are,
however, many individuals who have worked for the same
employer for many years. They have neither the experience
nor the skills required to face the "real world." They may suddenly feel that they have nothing to offer a new employer in
a highly competitive job market and they view themselves as
poor competitors. When their work was noncompetitive,
routinized, boring, and required few intellectual challenges,
these workers' capacity for autonomous decision-making became eroded. Such realizations inhibit individuals' perceptions of self-competence during a transitional period when self-

confidence is tied to success in achieving new employment.

Those having difficulty separating from a long-held job appear to be struggling with unresolved conflicts regarding attachment, separation, and loss. This is most frequently observed in workers who strongly identify with the workplace. Many companies use cultural, motivational, and economic strategies to stimulate loyalty, attachment, and identification. Organizations with high visibility and prestige also engender strong identification among their employees, and job loss results in an accompanying loss of status. Individuals with strong loyalty to their employer and attachment to their workplace will actively deny the upcoming event and engage in fantasies and wish-fulfilling ideas. These take the form of rumors that the situation will reverse itself and that the impending event will be averted. An individual who reacts in this way appears to be avoiding the psychological trauma that this separation and eventual loss will engender. This type of reaction postpones the displaced worker's confrontation with loss and, at the same time, inhibits that person's ability to resolve the separation process. The ensuing depression and paralysis that surface appear to be rooted in attachment conflicts.

In order to manage a successful transition, therefore, the individual's morale needs to be bolstered. The sooner an individual relinquishes the self-imposed stigma associated with job loss and resolves the conflicts surrounding this change, the more able that person is to make the transition. The more competent person will move into an action mode in a timely fashion. Persons who have a low self-image, however, are less able to mobilize their efforts towards new employment. This may be due to a number of factors. Job loss due to a collective event, such as a plant closure or mass layoff, is still responded to in a personalized manner. During a period of publicized high employment, however, the paradox of "job loss amid affluence" creates confusion in the victim that often results in self-blame and guilt. A factor affecting vulnerable individuals is the loss of the anchor that a stable work environment provides, especially for the longer-term worker. The feeling of the workplace as a "home" is particularly prevalent among those whose primary form of social interaction is at their job. Single persons, older workers with relatively few social contacts, and others with weak support systems outside of work are more likely to make the workplace the locus of their daily lives.

There are some workplaces that are highly socialized, that is, characterized by a greater density of interpersonal ties among co-workers (Roy, 1960). This is especially evident in work environments where the task itself requires cooperation and a high degree of collaboration, such as emergency service workers and commercial fishermen. Co-workers are able to maintain close-knit social ties also in work situations where the tasks require little attention and become "automatic," and where the noise levels are low enough so that conversation is possible. Warehouse workers, service employees, packers, and other manual workers are more likely to engage in frequent conversation, because their work requires limited concentration. Occupations that require highly developed social skills, such as flight attendants, sales personnel, and retail clerks, involve workers in ongoing interaction.

These highly social employees are at risk when job loss occurs and they are unsuccessful in finding new employment. They experience the "social void" that is created by such dislocation as an intense loss, since the work environment has been the primary source of fulfillment of their social needs. Their sense of loss can be compared to what many behavioral scientists have observed among those who have experienced residential displacement due to urban renewal (Fried, 1963; 1980), community relocation and forced migration (de Wet, 1988; Lumsden, 1975; Marris, 1974; Scudder & Colson, 1982; Trimble, 1980), or relocation after destruction caused by natural or manmade disasters (Erikson, 1976). The destruction of a community and the displacement of its residents is an acknowledged stressor, because of the shared perception of loss. Even though a workplace functions as a "community" for longer-term employees, it lacks the cohesiveness and the institutional base that can support these social relationships. Once the job ends, many workplace relationships can only be sustained with considerable effort. The effects on these workers are similar to those reported by disaster victims, including the sense of alienation, disorientation, pessimism about the future, depression, and other post-traumatic symptoms. Individuals who have experienced frequent job loss, either voluntarily or through repeated layoffs, appear to be less able to risk attachment to a workplace, to be less willing to develop cohesive relationships with co-workers, and to have more difficulty forming a positive, purposive view of new employment. The numbing effect, described as a symptom of post-traumatic stress disorders, and observed as a transitional state in the more highly traumatized displaced worker, seems to persist in the person who has had multiple experiences with job loss.

References

Ahr, P. R., Gorodezky, J. J., & Cho, D. W. (1981). Measuring the relationship of public psychiatric admissions to rising unemployment. *Hospital and Community Psychiatry, 32,* 398–401.

Alexander, J. C. (1987). Action and its environments. In J. C. Alexander, B. Giesen, R. Munch, & N. J. Smelser (Eds.), *The Macro-Micro Link.* Berkeley: University of California Press.

American Psychiatric Association (1987). *Diagnostic and Statistical Manual of Mental Disorders 3rd edition, Revised.* Washington, DC: American Psychiatric Association.

Ames, G. M., & Janes, C. R. (1987a). Anthropology and prevention in North America: An introduction. *Social Science and Medicine, 25,* 921–922.

Ames, G. M., & Janes, C. R. (1987b) Heavy and problem drinking in an American blue-collar population: Implications for prevention. *Social Science and Medicine, 25,* 949–960.

Anderson, C., & Stark, C. (1988). Psychosocial problems of job relocation: Preventive roles in industry, *Social Work, 33,* 38–41.

Antonovsky, A. (1979). *Health, Stress and Coping.* San Francisco: Jossey-Bass.

Antonovsky, A. (1987). *Unraveling the Mystery of Health.* San Francisco: Jossey-Bass.

Atkinson, T., Liem, R., & Liem, J. H. (1986). The social costs of unemployment: Implications for social support. *Journal of Health and Social Behavior, 27,* 317–331.

Audy, J. R. (1971). Measurement and diagnosis of health. In P. Shepard & D. McKinley (Eds.), *Environ-Mental.* Boston: Houghton-Mifflin.

Bakke, E. W. (1940). *Citizens Without Work.* New Haven, CT: Institute of Human Relations, Yale University Press.

Bandura, A. (1977). Self-efficacy: Towards a unifying theory of behavioral change. *Psychological Review, 84,* 191–215.

Bandura, A. (1982). Self-efficacy mechanism in human agency. *American Psychologist, 37,* 122–147.

Banks, M. H., & Jackson, P. R. (1982). Unemployment and risk of minor psychiatric disorder in young people: Cross-sectional and longitudinal evidence. *Psychological Medicine, 12,* 789–798.

Baum, A., Fleming, R., & Reddy, D. M. (1986). Unemployment stress: Loss of control, reactance and learned helplessness. *Social Science and Medicine, 22,* 509–516.

Becker, H. S. & Strauss, A. L. (1960). Careers, personality and adult socialization. In M. R. Stein, A. J. Vidich, & D. M. White (Eds.), *Identity and*

Anxiety: Survival of the Person in Mass Society. Glencoe, NY: The Free Press.

Beckett, J. O. (1988). Plant closings: How older workers are affected. *Social Work, 33,* 29–33.

Bendix, R. (1974). *Work and Authority in Industry.* Berkeley: University of California Press.

Berki, S. E., Lichtenstein, R. & Wyszewianski, L. (1984) Study of the health needs of the unemployed. American Public Health Association *Medical Care Section Newsletter* (October), 2.

Bloom-Feshbach, J., & Bloom-Feshbach, S. (1987). Introduction: Psychological separateness and experiences of loss. In J. Bloom-Feshbach & S. Bloom-Feshbach (Eds.), *The Psychology of Separation and Loss: Perspectives on Development, Life Transitions and Clinical Practice.* San Francisco: Jossey-Bass.

Bluestone, B. & Harrison, B. (1982). *The Deindustrialization of America: Plant Closings, Community Abandonment and the Dismantling of Basic Industry.* New York: Basic Books.

Boor, M. (1980). Relationships between unemployment rates and suicide rates in eight countries, 1962–1976. *Psychological Reports, 47,* 1095–1101.

Bowen, M. (1971) Family and family group therapy. In H. I. Kaplan & B. J. Shaddock (Eds.), *Comprehensive Group Psychotherapy.* Baltimore: Williams & Williams.

Bowen, M. (1978). *Family Therapy in Clinical Practice.* New York: Jason Aronson.

Bowlby, J. (1973). *Separation: Anxiety and Anger.* New York: Basic Books.

Bowlby, J. (1980). *Loss: Sadness and Depression.* New York: Basic Books.

Bowlby, J. (1982). *Attachment* (2d Ed.). New York: Basic Books.

Braddock, J. H., & McPartland, J. M. (1987). How minorities continue to be excluded from equal employment opportunities: Research on labor market and institutional barriers. *Journal of Social Issues, 43,* 5–39.

Braverman, H. (1974). *Labor and Monopoly Capital.* New York & London: Monthly Review Press.

Breed, W. (1963). Occupational mobility and suicide among white males. *American Sociological Review, 28,* 179–188.

Brenner, M. H. (1973). *Mental Illness and the Economy.* Cambridge: Harvard University Press.

Brenner, M. H. (1976). Estimating the social costs of economic policy: Implications for mental and physical health and criminal aggression. Report to the Congressional Research Service of the Library of Congress and Joint Economic Committee of Congress, Washington, DC: U. S. Government Printing Office.

Brenner, M. H. (1980). Industrialization and economic growth: Estimates of their effects on the health of populations. In M. H. Brenner, A. Mooney, & T. J. Nagy (Eds.), *Assessing the Contributions of the Social Sciences to Health.* Boulder, CO: Westview Press.

Brenner, M. H. (1987a). Economic change, alcohol consumption and heart disease mortality in nine industrialized countries. *Social Science and Medicine, 25,* 119–132.

Brenner, M. H. (1987b). Relationship of economic change to Swedish health and social well-being, 1950–1980. *Social Science and Medicine, 25,* 183–195.

Bronfenbrenner, U. (1979). *The Ecology of Human Development*. Cambridge: Harvard University Press.

Buraway, M. (1979). *Manufacturing Consent: Changes in the Labor Process under Monopoly Capitalism*. Chicago: University of Chicago Press.

Buss, T. F., & Redburn, F. S. (1981). *Shutdown at Youngstown: Public Policy for Mass Unemployment*. Albany, NY: State University of New York Press.

Buss, T. F., & Redburn, F. S. (1983) *Mass Unemployment: Plant Closings and Community Mental Health*. Beverly Hills, CA: Sage Publications.

Butler, R. (1975). *Why Survive? Being Old in America*. New York: Harper & Row.

Caplan, G. (1964). *Principles of Preventive Psychiatry*. New York: Basic Books.

Caplan, G. (1970). *Theory and Practice of Mental Health Consultation*. New York: Basic Books.

Caplovitz, D. (1979). *Making Ends Meet: How Families Cope with Inflation and Recession*. Beverly Hills, CA: Sage Publications.

Cartwright, D., & Zander, A. (Eds.) (1968). *Group Dynamics: Research and Theory* (3rd ed.). New York: Harper & Row.

Catalano, R., & Dooley, D. (1977). Economic predictors of depressed mood and stressful life events in a metropolitan community. *Journal of Health and Social Behavior, 18*, 292–307.

Catalano, R., & Dooley, D. (1979). Does economic change provoke or uncover behavioral disorder? A preliminary test. In L. Ferman & J. Gordus (Eds.), *Mental Health and the Economy*. Kalamazoo, MI: W. E. Upjohn Institute for Employment Research.

Cobb, S. (1974). Psychological changes in men whose jobs were abolished. *Journal of Psychosomatic Research, 18*, 245–258.

Cobb, S. & Kasl, S. V. (1977). *Termination: The Consequences of Job Loss*. (Report #76-1261). Cincinnati, OH: National Institute for Occupational Safety and Health, Behavioral Motivation Factors Research.

Coburn, D. (1978). Work and general psychological and physical well-being. *International Journal of Health Services, 8*, 415–435.

Cohler, B. J., & Stott, F. M. (1987). Separation, interdependence and social relations across the second half of life. In J. Bloom-Feshbach & S. Bloom-Feshbach (Eds.), *The Psychology of Separation and Loss: Perspectives on Development, Life Transitions and Clinical Practice*. San Francisco: Jossey-Bass.

de Wet, C. J. (1988). Stress and environmental change in the analysis of community relocation. *Human Organization, 47*, 180–187.

Dohrenwend, B. S., & Dohrenwend, B. P. (1974). *Stressful Life Events: Their Nature and Effects*. New York: John Wiley.

Drennen, J. (1988). Responding to industrial plant closings and the unemployed. *Social Work, 33*, 50–52.

Durkheim, E. (1952). *Suicide: A Study of Sociology* (Translated by J. A. Spaulding & C. Simpson). London: Routledge and Kegan Paul.

Durman, E. C. (1976). The role of self-help in service provision. *Journal of Applied Behavioral Science, 12*, 433–443.

Edwards, R. (1979). *Contested Terrain: The Transformation of the Workplace in The Twentieth Century*. New York: Basic Books.

Eisenberg, P. & Lazarsfeld, P. F. (1938). The psychological effects of unemployment. *Psychological Bulletin, 35*, 358–389.

Erikson, K. (1976). *Everything in Its Path: Destruction of Community in the Buffalo Creek Flood*. New York: Simon & Schuster.

Festinger, L. (1957). *A Theory of Cognitive Dissonance*. Stanford, CA: Stanford University Press.

Field, T. (1985). Attachment as psychobiological attunement: Being on the same wavelength. In M. Reite & T. Field (Eds.), *The Psychobiology of Attachment and Separation*. Orlando, FL: Academic Press.

Figley, C. R. (1988). Toward a field of traumatic stress. *Journal of Traumatic Stress, 1*, 3–16.

Fleming, R., Baum, A., Reddy, D., & Gatchel, R. J. (1984). Behavioral and biochemical effects of job loss and unemployment stress. *Journal of Human Stress, 10*, 12–17.

Folkman, S., & Lazarus, R. S. (1988). The relationship between coping and emotion: Implications for theory and research. *Social Science and Medicine, 26*, 309–317.

Frese, M. (1987). Alleviating depression in the unemployed: Adequate financial support, hope and early retirement. *Social Science and Medicine, 25*, 213–215.

Frese, M., & Mohr, G. (1987). Prolonged unemployment and depression in older workers: A longitudinal study of intervening variables. *Social Science and Medicine, 25*, 173–178.

Fried, M. (1963). Grieving for a lost home. In L. J. Duhl (Ed.), *The Urban Condition: People and Policy in the Metropolis*. New York: Basic Books.

Fried, M. (1980). Stress, strain and role adaptation: Conceptual issues. In G. V. Coehlo & P. I. Ahmed (Eds.), *Uprooting and Development*. New York: Plenum Press.

Friedson, E. (1970). *Profession of Medicine: A Study of the Sociology of Applied Knowledge*. New York: Harper & Row.

Gardner, H. (1983). *Frames of Mind: The Theory of Multiple Intelligences*. New York: Basic Books.

Gardner, H. (1984). The development of competence in culturally defined domains: a preliminary framework. In R. A. Shweder & R. A. LeVine (Eds.), *Culture Theory: Essays on Mind, Self and Emotion*. Cambridge, England: Cambridge University Press.

Garfield J. (1980). Alienated labor, stress and coronary disease. *International Journal of Health Services, 10*, 551–560.

Gilligan, C. (1982). *In a Different Voice: Psychological Theory and Women's Development*. Cambridge: Harvard University Press.

Glaser, B. G., & Strauss, A. L. (1967). *The Discovery of Grounded Theory*. Chicago: Aldine.

Goffman, E. (1959). *The Presentation of Self in Everyday Life*. New York: Doubleday.

Goffman, E. (1963). *Stigma: Notes on the Management of Spoiled Identity*. Englewood Cliffs, NJ: Prentice-Hall.

Goffman, E. (1967). *Interaction Ritual*. New York: Doubleday.

Goffman, E. (1971). *Relations in Public*. New York: Basic Books.

Gore, S. (1978). The effects of social support in moderating the health consequences of unemployment. *Journal of Health and Social Behavior, 19*, 557–565.

Haber, W., Ferman, L. A., & Hudson, J. R. (1963). *The Impact of Technological Change*. Kalamazoo, MI: W. E. Upjohn Institute for Employment Research.

Haney, C. A. (1979). Life events as a precursor of coronary heart disease. *Social Science and Medicine, 13A,* 119–126.

Hartmann, H. I. (1987). Changes in women's economic and family roles in: post World War II United States. In L. Beneria & C. Stimpson (Eds.), *Women, Households and Structural Transformation.* New Brunswick, NJ: Rutgers University Press.

Harwood, A. (Ed.) (1981). *Ethnicity and Medical Care.* Cambridge: Harvard University Press.

Haynes, S. G., Feilieb, M., Levine, S., Scotch, N., & Kannel, W. B. (1978). The relationship of psychological factors to coronary heart disease in the Framingham Study II: Prevalence of coronary heart disease. *American Journal of Epidemiology, 107* (5), 384–402.

Hochschild, A. R. (1983). *The Managed Heart: Commercialization of Human Feeling.* Berkeley: University of California Press.

Holmes, T. H., & Rahe, R. H. (1967). The social readjustment rating scale. *Journal of Psychosomatic Research, 11,* 213–218.

Hurst, M. W., Jenkins, C. D., & Rose, R. M. (1976). The relationship of psychological stress to onset of medical illness. *Annual Review of Medicine, 27.*

Jacobson, D. (1987). Models of stress and meanings of unemployment: Reactions to job loss among technical professionals. *Social Science and Medicine, 24,* 13–21.

Jahoda, M. (1979). The impact of unemployment in the 1930's and the 1970's. *Bulletin of the British Psychological Society, 32,* 309–314.

Jahoda, M., Lazarsfeld, P. F., & Zeisel, H. (1971). *Marienthal: the Sociography of an Unemployment Community.* Chicago: Aldine-Atherton.

Joelson, L. & Wahlquist, L. (1987). The psychological meaning of job insecurity and job loss: Results of a longitudinal study. *Social Science and Medicine, 25,* 179–182.

Kanter, R. M. (1977). *Men and Women of the Corporation.* New York: Basic Books.

Kasl, S. V., & Cobb, S. (1979). Some mental health consequences of plant closing and job loss. In L. A. Ferman & J. P. Gordus (Eds.), *Mental Health and the Economy.* Kalamazoo, MI: W. E. Upjohn Institute for Employment Research.

Kasl, S. V., & Cobb, S., (1982). Variability of stress effects among men experiencing job loss. In L. Goldberger & S. Breznitz (Eds.), *Handbook of Stress: Theoretical and Clinical Aspects.* New York: Free Press.

Kasl, S., Gore, S., & Cobb, S. (1975). The experience of losing a job: Reported change in health symptoms and illness behavior. *Psychosomatic Medicine, 37,* 106–122.

Katz, A. H., & Bender, E. I. (1976). *The Strength in Us: Self-Help Groups in the Modern World.* New York: Franklin Watts.

Kaufman, H. G. (1982). *Professionals in Search of Work: Coping with the Stress of Job Loss and Underemployment.* New York: John Wiley.

Kelvin, P., & Jarrett, J. E. (1985). *Unemployment: Its Social Psychological Effects.* London: Cambridge University Press.

Kessler, R. C., House, J. S., & Turner, J. B. (1987). Unemployment and health in a community sample. *Journal of Health and Social Behavior, 28,* 51–59.

Ketterer, R. F. (1981). *Consultation and Education in Mental Health: Problems and Prospects*. Newbury Park, CA: Sage Publications.

King, C. (1982). *The Social Impacts of Mass Layoff*. Ann Arbor, MI: Center for Research on Social Organization, University of Michigan (mimeo).

Kohn, M. L. (1977). *Class and Conformity* (2nd ed.). Chicago: University of Chicago Press.

Kohn, M. L. (1980). Job complexity and adult personality. In N. J. Smelser & E. H. Erikson (Eds.), *Themes of Love and Work in Adulthood*. Cambridge: Harvard University Press.

Kolb, D. A. (1984). *Experiential Learning: Experience as the Source of Learning and Development*. Englewood Cliffs, NJ: Prentice-Hall.

Komarovsky, M. (1940). *The Unemployed Man and His Family: The Effect of Unemployment upon the Status of the Man in 59 Families*. New York: Dryden Press.

Kreitler, S., & Kreitler, H. (1988). Trauma and anxiety: The cognitive approach. *Journal of Traumatic Stress, 1*, 35–56.

Kubler-Ross, E. (1969). *On Death and Dying*. New York: Macmillan.

LaRocco, J. M., House, J. S., & French, J. R. P. (1980). Social support, occupational stress, and health. *Journal of Health and Social Behavior, 21*, 202–218.

Lefkovitz, R., & Withorn, A. (Eds.). (1986). *For Crying Out Loud: Women and Poverty in the United States*. New York: The Pilgrim Press.

Lerner, M. (1985). *Occupational Stress Groups and the Psychodynamics of the World of Work*. Oakland, CA: Institute for Labor and Mental Health.

Lerner, M. (1986). *Surplus Powerlessness*. Oakland, CA: Institute for Labor and Mental Health.

Levinson, D. J. (1979). *The Seasons of a Man's Life*. New York: Knopf.

Levinson, D. J. (1986). A conception of adult development. *American Psychologist, 41*, 3–13.

Liem, R. (1983). Beyond economics: The health costs of unemployment. *Health and Medicine, 2*, 3–9.

Liem, R. (1987). The psychological costs of unemployment: A comparison of findings and definitions. *Social Research, 54*, 319–353.

Liem, R., Atkinson, T., & Liem, J. (1982). The work and unemployment project: Personal and family effects of job loss. Unpublished paper, Dept. of Psychology, University of Massachusetts at Boston.

Little, C. B. (1976). Technical-professional unemployment: Middle-class adaptability to personal crisis. *The Sociological Quarterly, 17*, 262–274.

Lumsden, D. P. (1975). Towards a systems model of stress: Feedback from an anthropological study of Ghana's Upper Volta River Project. In I. Sarason & C. Speilberger (Eds.), *Stress and Anxiety*, Vol. 2, New York: Hemisphere/Wiley.

Lutz, C. (1985). Depression and the translation of emotional worlds. In A. Kleinman & B. Good (Eds.), *Culture and Depression: Studies in the Anthropology and Cross-Cultural Psychiatry of Affect and Disorder*. Berkeley: University of California Press.

Mandler, G. (1984). *Mind and Body: Psychology of Emotion and Stress*. New York: Norton.

Marris, P. (1974). *Loss and Change.* London: Routledge & Kegan Paul.

Marris, P.(1980). The uprooting of meaning. In G. V. Coehlo & P. I. Ahmed (Eds.), *Uprooting and Development.* New York: Plenum Press.

Marris, P. (1982) Attachment and society. In C. M. Parkes & J. Stevenson-Hinde (Eds.), *The Place of Attachment in Human Behavior.* New York: Basic Books.

Maslow, A. H. (1987). *Motivation and Personality* (3rd ed.). New York: Harper & Row.

McClelland, D. C. (1961). *The Achieving Society.* Princeton, NJ: Van Nostrand.

Miller, J. G. (1978). *Living Systems.* New York: McGraw-Hill.

Minuchin, S. (1974). *Families and Family Therapy.* Cambridge: Harvard University Press.

Mitchell, J. T. (1983). When disaster strikes . . . The critical incident debriefing process. *Journal of Emergency Medical Services, 8,* 36–39.

Mitchell, J. T. (1985). Healing the helper. In *Role Stressors and Supports for Emergency Workers.* Rockville, MD: National Institute of Mental Health.

Mitchell, R. E., Billings, A. G., & Moos, R. H. (1982). Social support and well-being: Implications for prevention programs. *Journal of Primary Prevention, 3,* 77–98.

Morris, J. B., Kovacs, M., Beck, A., & Wolffe, A. (1974). Notes towards an epidemiology of urban suicide. *Comprehensive Psychiatry, 14,* 537–547.

Newman, K. S. (1988). *Falling from Grace: The Experience of Downward Mobility in the American Middle Class.* New York: The Free Press.

Nichols, M. P. (1986). *Turning Forty in the Eighties.* New York: Simon & Schuster.

O'Connor, J. (1987). *The Meaning of Crisis: A Theoretical Introduction.* Oxford and New York: Basil Blackwell.

Parkes, C. M. (1982). Attachment and the prevention of mental disorders. In C. M. Parkes & J. Stevenson-Hinde (Eds.), *The Place of Attachment in Human Behavior.* New York: Basic Books.

Parnes, H. S., & King, R. (1977). Middle-aged job losers. *Industrial Gerontology, 4,* 77–95.

Perlin, L. I., & Lieberman, M. A. (1979). Social sources of emotional stress. In R. G. Simmons (Ed.), *Research in Community and Mental Health.* Greenwich, CT: JAI.

Petrovich, S. B., & Gewirtz, J. L. (1985). The attachment learning process and its relation to cultural and biological evolution: Proximate and ultimate considerations. In M. Reite & T. Field (Eds.), *The Psychobiology of Attachment and Separation.* Orlando, FL: Academic Press.

Piotrkowski, C. S., & Gornick, L. K. (1987). Effects of work-related separations on children and families. In J. Bloom-Feshbach & S. Bloom-Feshbach (Eds.), *The Psychology of Separation and Loss: Perspectives on Development, Life Transitions and Clinical Practice.* San Francisco: Jossey-Bass.

Piven, F. F., & Cloward, R. A. (1971). *Regulating the Poor: The Functions of Public Welfare.* New York: Pantheon.

Piven, F. F., & Cloward, R. A. (1977). *Poor People's Movements: Why They Succeed, How They Fail.* New York: Random House.

Popay, J. (1982). Responding to unemployment at a local level. Paper presented at the Workshop of Health Policy in Relation to Unemployment in the Community, December, 1982, Nuffield Center, Leeds, England.

Powell, E. (1958). Occupation, status and suicide: Towards a redefinition of anomie. *American Sociological Review, 23,* 131–139.

Powell, D. H., & Driscoll, P. J. (1973). Middle-class professionals face unemployment. *Society, 10,* 18–26.

Rahe, R. H., & Lind, E. (1971). Psychosocial factors and sudden cardiac death: A pilot study. *Journal of Psychosomatic Research, 15,* 14–19.

Rahe, R. H., Romo, M., Bennett, L., & Siltanen, P. (1976). *Subject's Recent Life Changes and Myocardial Infarction in Helsinki.* San Diego, CA: U. S. Navy Medical Neuropsychiatric Research Unit.

Rayman, P. M. & Bluestone, B. (1982a). *Out of Work: The Consequences of Unemployment in the Hartford Aircraft Industry.* Final Report (Research Grant No. MH 33251). Boston: Social Welfare Research Institute, Boston College.

Rayman, P. M., & Bluestone, B. (1982b). *The Private and Social Response to Job Loss: A Metropolitan Study.* Rockville, MD: National Institute of Mental Health.

Reite, M. & Capitanio, J. P. (1985). On the nature of social separation and social attachment. In M. Reite & T. Field (Eds.), *The Psychobiology of Attachment and Separation.* Orlando, FL: Academic Press.

Ries, R. W. (1983). *Americans Assess Their Health: United States, 1978* (DHHS Publication No. PHS 83-1570, Series 10, Number 142). Hyattsville, MD: National Cennter for Health Statistics.

Revicki, D. A., & May, H. J. (1985). Occupational stress, social support and depression. *Health Psychology, 4,* 61–77.

Root, K. (1979). *Perspectives for Community and Organizations on Job Closings and Job Dislocation.* Ames, IA: Iowa University Press.

Rosow, I. (1974). *Socialization to Old Age.* Berkeley: University of California Press.

Roy, D. F. (1960). "Banana time" job satisfaction and informal interaction. *Human Organization, 18,* 158–169.

Rubin, L. B. (1976). *Worlds of Pain: Life in the Working Class Family.* New York: Basic Books.

Rutter, M. (1987). Psychosocial resilience and protective mechanisms. *American Journal of Orthopsychiatry, 57,* 316–331.

Sainsbury, P. (1955). *Suicide in London: An Ecological Study.* Maudsley Monograph No. 1, London: Chapman and Hall.

Sanborn, D. E., Sanborn, C. J., & Cimbolic, P. (1974). Occupation and suicide. *Diseases of the Nervous System, 35,* 7–12.

Schaps, S. (1983). Building a community unemployment union. *Health and Medicine, 2,* 16–17.

Schein, E. H. (1978). *Career Dynamics: Matching Individual and Organizational Needs.* Reading, MA: Addison-Wesley.

Schein, E. H. (1985). *Organizational Culture and Leadership.* San Francisco: Jossey-Bass.

Scudder, T. & Colson, E. (1982). From welfare to development: A conceptual framework for the analysis of dislocated people. In A. Hansen & A. Oliver-Smith (Eds.), *Involuntary Migration and Resettlement.* Boulder, CO: Westview Press.

Sennett, R., & Cobb, J. (1972). *The Hidden Injuries of Class.* New York: Random House.

Shepherd, D. M., & Barraclough, B. M. (1980). Work and suicide: An empirical investigation. *British Journal of Psychiatry, 136,* 469–478.

Sloate, A. (1969). *Termination: The Closing at Baker Plant.* New York: Bobbs-Merrill.

Smith, J. (1984). The paradox of women's poverty: Wage-earning women and economic transformation. *Signs, 10*(2), 291–310.

Stone, J., & Kieffer, C. (1984). *Pre-Layoff Intervention: A Response to Unemployment.* Ann Arbor: Michigan Department of Mental Health and Industrial Development Division, Institute of Science and Technology, The University of Michigan.

Taber, T. D., Walsh, J. T., & Cooke, R. A. (1979). Developing a community-based program for reducing the impact of a plant closing. *Journal of Applied Behavioral Science, 15,* 133–155.

Theorell, T., & Rahe, R. H. (1971). Psychosocial factors and myocardial infarction I: An inpatient study in Sweden. *Journal of Psychosomatic Research, 15,* 25–32.

Thompson, W. H. (1983). Working together: Health care providers in their communities. *Health and Medicine, 2,* 11–12.

Trimble, J. E. (1980). Forced migration: Its impact on shaping coping strategies. In G. V. Coehlo & P. I. Ahmed (Eds.), *Uprooting and Development.* New York: Plenum Press.

Vaillant, G. (1977). *Adaptation to Life.* Boston: Little, Brown.

Vingerhoets, A. J. J. M., & Marcelissen, F. H. G. (1988). Stress research: Its present status and issues for future developments. *Social Science and Medicine, 26,* 279–291.

Wallace, A. F. C. (1957). Mazeway disintegration: The individual's perception of socio-cultural disorganization. *Human Organization, 16,* 23–27.

Wallerstein, J. S., & Kelly, J. B. (1980). *Surviving the Break-up: How Children and Parents Cope with Divorce.* New York: Basic Books.

Wallston, B. S., Alagna, S. W., DeVellis, B. McE., & DeVellis, R. F. (1983). Social support and physical health. *Health Psychology, 2,* 367–391.

Warr, P. (1984). Job loss, unemployment and psychological well-being. In V. L. Allen & E. Van de Vleit (Eds.), *Role Transitions: Explorations and Explanations.* New York: Plenum Press.

Warr, P., & Jackson, P. (1987). Adapting to the unemployed role: A longitudinal investigation. *Social Science and Medicine, 25,* 1219–1224.

Weiner, H. (1974). The concept of stress in the light of studies on disaster, unemployment and loss: A critical analysis. In B. S. Dohrenwend & B. P. Dohrenwend (Eds.), *Stressful Life Events: Their Nature and Effects.* New York: John Wiley.

Weiss, R. S. (1975). *Marital Separation.* New York: Basic Books.

White, R. W. (1979). Competence as an aspect of personal growth. In M. W. Kent & J. E. Rolf (Eds.), *Social Competence in Children.* Hanover: University Press of New England.

Whyte, W. F. (1969). *Organizational Behavior.* Homewood, IL: Irwin/Dorsey.

Young, M., & Willmott, P. (1957). *Family and Kinship in East London.* London: Routledge & Kegan Paul.

Young, M., & Willmott, P. (1973). *The Symmetrical Family.* New York: Pantheon.

Name Index

197

Subject Index

200

About the Authors

CARL A. MAIDA, PH.D., is Assistant Research Anthropologist, School of Public Health, University of California, Los Angeles.

NORMA S. GORDON, M.A., is a specialist in program consultation, training, and resources development in the human services field.

NORMAN L. FARBEROW, PH.D., is Co-Director of The Suicide Prevention Center, 1041 South Menlo Avenue, Los Angeles, California.

Printed and bound by CPI Group (UK) Ltd, Croydon, CR0 4YY

17/10/2024

01775688-0019